# Ramayana for Children

**Aruna Trivedi** has worked in an international consultancy firm. She has widely travelled both in India—including pilgrimages—and abroad. Her book *Ramayan: Samay Ki Kasauti Per* is widely read.

# Ramayana for Children

## ARUNA TRIVEDI

RUPA

Published by
Rupa Publications India Pvt. Ltd 2018
7/16, Ansari Road, Daryaganj
New Delhi 110002

*Sales Centres:*
Allahabad Bengaluru Chennai
Hyderabad Jaipur Kathmandu
Kolkata Mumbai

Copyright © Aruna Trivedi 2018

The views and opinions expressed in this book are the author's own and the facts are as reported by him which have been verified to the extent possible, and the publishers are not in any way liable for the same.

All rights reserved.
No part of this publication may be reproduced, transmitted, or stored in a retrieval system, in any form or by any means, electronic, mechanical, photocopying, recording or otherwise, without the prior permission of the publisher.

ISBN: 978-93-5333-266-2

First impression 2018

10 9 8 7 6 5 4 2 3 1

The moral right of the author has been asserted.

Printed by Nutech Print Services, Faridabad

This book is sold subject to the condition that it shall not, by way of trade or otherwise, be lent, resold, hired out, or otherwise circulated, without the publisher's prior consent, in any form of binding or cover other than that in which it is published.

*To my grandchildren*

# Contents

The Birth of Rama / 1

Sita's Swyamvar / 13

Journey to the Forest / 25

The Abduction of Sita / 41

The Slaying of Vali / 54

The Lankan Inferno / 76

The Battle of Lanka I / 106

The Battle of Lanka II / 130

The Coronation of Lord Rama / 158

Sita's Exile / 161

The Ashwamedh Yagn / 165

The Journey to the Heavens / 179

# The Birth of Rama

In Treta Yug, the Kingdom of Ayodhya was ruled by King Dasharatha. He belonged to the Raghu clan of the Sun Dynasty. Sage Vasishtha was the chief priest of Ayodhya.

Dasharatha had three most important queens. The eldest, Kaushalya, was from Kosala. His second queen was Sumitra from Magadh Pradesh and the third and youngest one, Kaikeyi, was from Kekaya Pradesh. She was very beautiful, brave, ambitious, diplomatic, and a good warrior. She also accompanied the King in war.

Dasharatha was very fond of his third queen and she also wanted to be with him. Both of them had common interests and their personal traits were also similar. So, she had more influence over the King.

Once, Dasharatha helped Lord Indra during a war. At that time, Kaikeyi saved Dasharatha's life, and as a reward, he granted her two boons. She said, 'I choose to ask for these boons when I desire.'

As Dasharatha grew old, the thought of being without children began to bother him. He worried about the successor of the vast empire. Dasharatha consulted his priests over this matter and took their advice. He organized many yagns and observed fasts but all in vain.

Dasharatha's finance minister and friend, Sumantra, recommended the Putrakameshti Yagn to the King. He said, 'King Rompad has a daughter named Shanta, and her husband is Sage Rishyasringa. You should go to King Rompad and adopt the couple as your daughter- and son-in-law respectively, and bring them to Ayodhya. If you are able to perform the yagn under the supervision of this sage, you will be blessed with a son.'

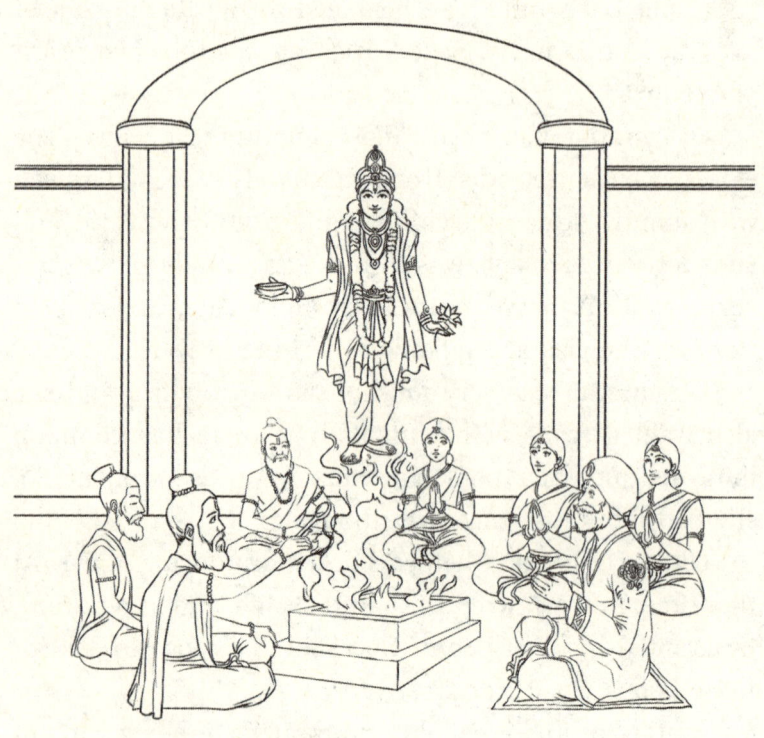

Dasharatha, along with his queens, went to King Rompad. He brought the couple to Ayodhya and the rishi performed the yagn. A man emerged from the sacrificial fire. He announced that he was the messenger of Lord Brahma and had brought with him a bowl of *kheer* or divine rice pudding. He told Dasharatha to give it to his queens. Dasharatha gave half of the pudding to Kaikeyi, whom he loved the most, and the other half to Kaushalya, as she was the eldest queen. The two queens shared half of each of their shares with Sumitra.

In due course, Kaushalya gave birth to Rama—the eldest son; Kaikeyi gave birth to Bharata; Sumitra gave birth to Lakshmana and Shatrughana—twins, and the youngest of all the sons.

The special attachment among the princes and their characteristics arose from the way the divine pudding was distributed among the three queens. Rama and Bharata were look-alikes and were blessed with a dark complexion. Lakshmana and Shatrughana, on the other hand, looked similar and were fair-skinned.

The princes were very fond of each other and roamed around the kingdom in pairs—Rama with Lakshmana and Bharata with Shatrughana. With the onset of adolescence, they left for Sage Vasishtha's ashram for education in scriptures and warfare.

Janaka, the ruler of Mithila, was a noble and pious king. His kingdom was going through difficult times as it had been hit by famine. He opened his warehouses and granaries to his people, so that no one died of hunger in his kingdom. He was worried that after some time the godowns would run out of grains. What would happen then? He made every effort to overcome the famine, but all was in vain. He took advice from the saints and priests of the kingdom to overcome this issue.

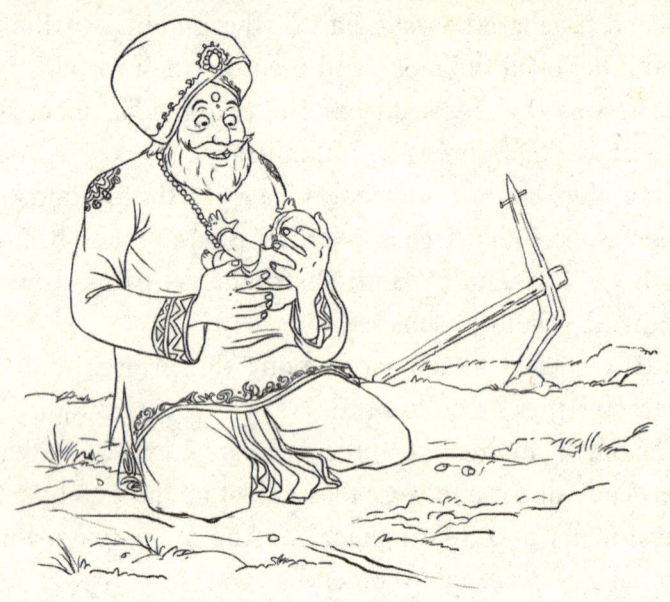

The chief priest of Mithila and son of Ahilya, Satananda, discussed the issue with other priests of the kingdom and arrived at a decision. He suggested that if the king tilled the fields with a golden plough, the land would yield plenty of crops. King Janaka did as told for the welfare of his people.

While ploughing the field, he found a tiny baby girl in an earthen pot. Janaka and his wife Sunaina took her to their palace, where she was brought up as their own child. The famine ended and Mithila prospered once again. Since Janaka had found the girl in a furrow of a ploughed field, she was regarded as the daughter of the Earth Goddess. Thus, she was named Sita. After Sita, Janaka was blessed with a daughter whom he named Urmila, and a son, Laxminidhi.

It is believed that whenever righteousness is challenged and non-believers take over, God comes into the world as an avatar to protect the virtuous and punish the sinners. Lord Vishnu took birth as Rama during a similar crisis. A few years after Rama's birth, Lord Shiva, along with a monkey, paid a visit to Sage Vasishtha. He said, 'This monkey is Hanuman. Lord Rama has taken birth. Goddess Lakshmi has been born as Sita to Janaka, the King of Mithila. You and Hanuman, with the help of Sage Vishwamitra, will play a crucial role in uniting Rama and Sita.'

Sage Vishwamitra's ashram, Siddhashrama, was located near a dense forest called Tadaka Van. The ashram was named so because Lord Vishnu had attained *siddhi*, or mystical power, here. Ravana, the King of Lanka, had established pickets at different places in this forest. From these pickets, Ravana controlled the rishis in the hermitages. He deployed soldiers at these pickets and instructed them to prevent any kind of sacrifice or prayer in these areas. Ravana feared that through these prayers the rishis might become more powerful than him. The soldiers abided by these orders and disrupted any kind of prayer, obeisance and penance by these rishis.

A picket of Ravana's soldiers, under the command of the demoness Tadaka, was located close by. She resided here with her son, Maricha, and companion, Subahu. Tadaka was basically a *yakshini*, or demigod, who was cursed to become a demoness. The demons were a nuisance and caused hindrances during yagns by throwing blood and flesh at the yagnakunda.

Meanwhile, Vishwamitra had organized a big yagn and it was time for *poornahuti* or the final oblation. His only fear was that the yagn could be destroyed by the demons like all the other times. Despite being a good warrior, Vishwamitra could not have left the yagn; nor could he get angry and begin fighting the demons. This was the rule of performing any yagn.

Suddenly, it occurred to Vishwamitra that it is a king's duty to help his people when in need, during worship, to gain knowledge, earn wealth and so on. He set off to Ayodhya for help. When the rishi reached Ayodhya, King Dasharatha was humbled by his presence and welcomed him warmly. Ensuring that the sage was comfortable, the King asked him the purpose of his visit. Before listening to what Vishwamitra wanted, Dasharatha assured him whatsoever he desired would be granted.

Vishwamitra informed him that he had performed a great yagn. After its completion, he needed to perform the final rites. Two demons, who could change their forms, were trying to prevent him from completing the yagn. He explained that the rishis were not allowed to even curse them in the midst of their worship. He requested Dasharatha to allow Rama and Lakshmana to go with him to eliminate the demons.

Dasharatha became reluctant on hearing the sage's request. He thought that the princes were still too young to engage in a battle with demons. He did not want to part with Rama especially, as he was his favourite, and send him on such dangerous missions. Dasharatha offered Vishwamitra his entire army. He told him that if the sage desired, the King would himself lead the battle, but he wouldn't allow Rama and Lakshmana to do so.

Vishwamitra became furious when the King refused to send his sons on the mission. He said, 'First, you promised to fulfil any desire and now when I asked for it, you are going back on your word. This is not what the Raghukul dynasty's tradition dictates. If you cannot send Rama and Lakshmana with me, you can refuse straight away. I will go back without any help from you.'

Vasishtha intervened and tried to reason with Dasharatha by telling him that a King would never want the standards of the Raghu clan to fall. Vasishtha explained to Dasharatha that he was born as a human embodiment of dharma in his clan and he should not allow emotions to influence his decisions. It was his responsibility to send Rama and Lakshmana with Vishwamitra to the forest. He also added that it did not matter how experienced Rama and Lakshmana were in warfare. The demons would not be able to withstand his sons as long as Vishwamitra was with them.

On their way back to Siddhashrama, Vishwamitra narrated Tadaka's story to Rama and Lakshmana—her birth, marriage and what led her to become a demoness. He told Rama that he must kill her and should not hesitate to do so because she is a woman, as the Sanatan Dharma does not allow a king to kill a woman except to protect his people.

After listening to Vishwamitra's advice, Rama drew his bow and a loud twang reverberated through the forest. Tadaka appeared in front of them. Lakshmana cut off her nose and ears and she growled in pain and anger. She raised a cloud of dust so thick that it was difficult to see through. Rama drew a sound-sensing arrow and released it in the direction of Tadaka, killing her.

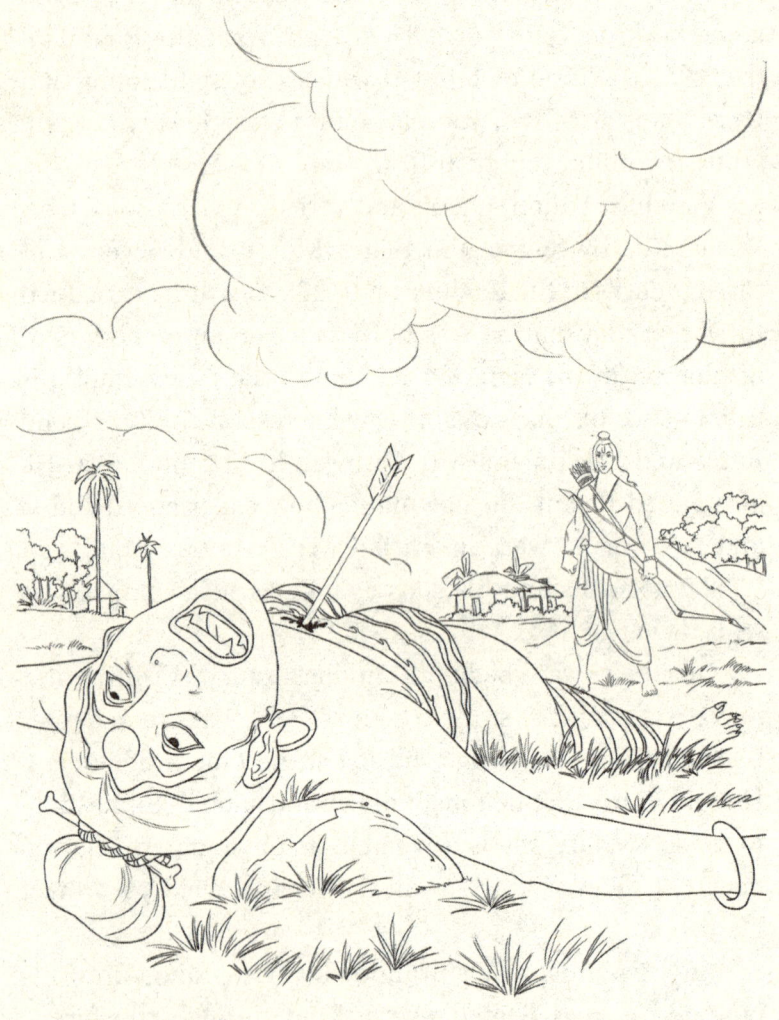

After slaying Tadaka, they continued on their path and Vishwamitra taught Rama and Lakshmana ways to live without food and sleep in a forest for a long period and still remain energetic. He gave Rama and Lakshmana about sixty divine weapons. He also taught them how to use them.

In this way, Rama and Lakshmana had two gurus (teachers)—Vasishtha and Vishwamitra. Vasishtha taught them the art of politics, warfare, yog and the vedas. Vishwamitra taught them science and technicalities—the use of divine weapons.

After learning the use of these weapons, they reached Siddhashrama. It was located at the confluence of river Ganga and river Saryu. This was the place where Lord Shiva used to meditate. It was this place where he had burnt Kamadev to ashes with his third eye.

Vishwamitra started the yagn with Rama and Lakshmana keeping guard. Six days passed peacefully. On the seventh day, Maricha came to the ashram. Rama used a weapon which does not kill but throws the enemy thousands of miles away. One after the other, the demons were killed and Vishwamitra was able to complete the yagn.

Sita was brought up in the palace of King Janaka with a lot of affection and care. She was very beautiful. Eventually, Janaka thought it was time to get her married. Since Sita was described as the daughter of the earth, her peculiar birth aroused doubts in the minds of her suitors and the respectable families were unwilling to get their sons married to her. However, those who were interested were kings like Ravana and Banasur, and Janaka was not keen on getting Sita married to them. So he turned down their proposals.

Janaka had a bow which belonged to the great warrior saint Parashurama. The bow was originally given to Parashurama by Lord Shiva. Legend has it that when Parashurama avenged the death of his father, he killed many Kshatriya warriors. It is also believed that he wiped out the entire Kshatriya race from the face of the earth twenty-one times. In the end, he relinquished his weapons, including the bow, and took up yoga.

Parashurama had found Janaka to be the most suitable person for the bow's custody. The bow was so heavy that no one could lift it. It was locked up in a room on a platform which had four wheels. The weight of the bow made the platform impossible to move. No one, except Sita, was permitted to enter the room to clean it.

One day, Janaka noticed that Sita, very casually, lifted the bow with one hand and wiped the place where it rested. Then, she effortlessly placed it right back. Janaka understood that Sita had divine powers. He then decided to find a suitable match for her.

Janaka thought of organizing the Dhanush Yagn, as he knew that no ordinary person was capable of lifting the bow (*dhanush*). He declared that the person who lifts the bow and strings it will wed Sita.

Invitations were immediately sent out and one of them reached Vishwamitra's ashram too. He decided to go to Mithila with Rama and Lakshmana to attend the *swayamvar* (the ceremony of choosing one's own husband). As they were approaching Milthila, they came across an abandoned ashram. Rama wondered why the ashram was so desolate. Vishwamitra, along with Rama and Lakshmana, entered it.

Vishwamitra explained that it used to be the ashram of Sage Gautama Maharishi. He, along with his wife Ahilya and their five-year-old son Satananda, used to live here. There were other saints too who lived with him in the ashram. Princes and children from royal families were sent here for education. Everyone lived happily until one day when Gautama invited the gods for a yagn. When Lord Indra saw Ahilya, he was bewitched by her beauty.

The next morning, when Gautama had gone to the river for ablutions, Lord Indra transformed himself into Gautama. According to Valmiki, when Indra entered the cottage, Ahilya could not see through the disguise and accepted his advances. Meanwhile, when Gautama returned home, he saw Indra leaving his cottage in his guise. Gautama understood what had happened and cursed Ahilya and Indra, and she would only be relinquished from the curse by Lord Rama. Sage Gautama left for the Himalayas to meditate. All the other sages and students left that place and joined other ashrams.

Rama was furious after listening to this story. He was disappointed with Sage Gautama's reaction to the episode. As such, he touched Ahilya with affection and she was transformed into her real form.

Vishwamitra, along with Rama and Lakshmana, started for Mithila once again. During the course of their journey,

Vishwamitra apprised Rama on the history of Shiva's Dhanush and how it had reached Janaka. He also taught him how to use it.

# Sita's Swyamvar

Vishwamitra, along with Rama and Lakshmana, reached Mithila. The kingdom is also called Janakapuri after its king, Janaka. Similarly, Sita is also called Janaki, as she is the daughter of Janaka.

When the news of Vishwamitra's arrival reached Janaka, he personally went to welcome him with his chief priest Satananda. After exchanging pleasantries, Janaka enquired about the princes accompanying him.

Vishwamitra introduced him to both the princes. Janaka made appropriate arrangements for their stay and comfort. Later in the evening, with the permission of the rishi, Rama and Lakshmana went to explore the city. Wherever they went, the people were very happy to see them. They were impressed by their appearance and mannerisms. Even though they seemed delicate, the people thought that Rama would make the best suitor for Sita. The women found them more handsome than the gods. Vishnu had four hands. Shiva had a fierce appearance. Therefore, none of the gods could be compared to Rama. The people of Mithila also came to know that Rama and Lakshmana had helped Vishwamitra kill the demons. But they still wondered if Rama would be able to lift and string the bow.

Rama and Lakshmana reached the venue where the Dhanush Yagn was to be held. It was a large arena with seating arrangements for different statures of men and women. There was a vedi at the centre. Around it, there were thrones made of gold for kings and princes participating in the ceremony. A person was deputed to show Rama and Lakshmana around. The two princes got so engrossed in the beauty of the place that they lost track of time. It was quite late, and they hurried back to their guest house.

The next morning, Rama and Lakshmana woke up early. They finished their chores and went to Vishwamitra. After offering him salutations, they sought his permission to go to the garden to fetch flowers for the morning prayer.

The garden was very pleasant. There were plants and vines laden with flowers all around. The chirping of birds set a romantic tone to the ambiance. At the centre of the garden, there was a pond full of beautiful lotus flowers. There was also a temple in the garden.

Coincidentally, Sita had also come to the temple with her friends or *sakhi*s, after plucking flowers from the garden and taking a dip in the pond. Sita offered the flowers to Devi Parvati and prayed for a suitable groom for herself. One of her friends was roaming in the garden. She saw both the princes there. She immediately came to Sita and told her about the two princes roaming in the garden. They were probably the same princes who had arrived the previous day with Vishwamitra. Out of curiosity, Sita eagerly walked towards the garden, where Rama and Lakshmana were plucking flowers. Hearing the sweet tinkle of bangles and anklets, or *payal*s, they knew that the girls were approaching. Rama peered in the direction of the sound and saw a very beautiful girl. She was so beautiful that

Rama forgot to bat his eyelids. He told Lakshmana that she seemed to be princess Sita for whom this ceremony was being organized. Sita also looked around to spot the princes and saw them standing in the shadow of a tree. She was charmed by Rama's personality and closed her eyes, slightly abashed. Rama and Lakshmana stepped out of the shadow. Sita's friend told her to open her eyes. Sita opened her eyes and saw Rama.

Her *sakhi*s hurried Sita as her mother was expecting her and might get angry due to the delay. Sita followed her friends. However, the toughness of the Shiva Dhanush began to bother her. She again went to the temple and prayed to Goddess Parvati. She said, 'Devi Maa, you know what I desire. When Rama picks up the Dhanush, please make it lighter, as this delicate and young prince might not be able to string it.' At that very moment, a garland fell from the idol onto Sita's hand. She understood that Parvati had granted her wish. She went back to the palace happily and Rama and Lakshmana also headed back to their Guru. They narrated the incident to Vishwamitra.

The next day, Janaka asked Satananda to fetch the rishi and the princes. Vishwamitra called Rama and Lakshmana and started for the venue.

Vishwamitra praised the ceremonial site and Janaka was very pleased. The suitors had different feelings about Rama and Lakshmana. Some of them thought Sita would select the handsome prince even if he failed to lift and string the bow. Others thought, even if Rama succeeded, they would not let him marry Sita.

Janaka called Sita to the ceremonial site. Sita came and

sat at the place designated for her. The courtiers repeatedly praised Janaka.

One by one, the kings tried their luck with the bow but were unsuccessful. They felt humiliated and went back to their seats. Some did not even dare to try their hands at it. Ravana and Banasur too had come. They just walked around the bow, and after offering their salutations, went back to their seats. Thousands of kings tried to lift the bow and string it but failed.

Janaka was saddened and angry. He said, 'It seems Lord Brahma has not created a man powerful enough to string the bow, and hold my daughter's hand in matrimony. It seems that the earth is starving and has no real warriors. Had I known this, I would not have taken the vow. Now, all of you can go back to your homes. It seems like Sita will remain unmarried.'

Listening to this, Lakshmana rose from his seat and declared, 'When someone from the Raghukul is present in an assembly, no one should demean the audience, especially when Shree Rama is one of them. I can lift the universe like a ball and smash it like an earthen pot; I can break the Sumeru Mountain. I can lift this bow like a toy and run for aeons.'

Janaka got embarrassed after listening to Lakshmana. Rama signalled Lakshmana to sit down. Then Vishwamitra said to Rama, 'Get up, go ahead, lift the bow and break it.'

Sita's mother Sunaina was perplexed by his words. She asked her friends why no one was telling Vishwamitra to desist from this foolhardy act. She said, 'This bow is very heavy. Ravana and Banasur did not even dare to lift it. This prince is very delicate. How can he do the impossible?'

Her friend told her that she should not estimate a warrior by his appearance. 'Agastaya rishi, born from a pitcher, could drink all the seas' water. A small ray of sunlight lightens up the three worlds. A mahout is able to control an elephant with the help of a small trident or *ankush*. So, set aside your apprehension; Rama will be able to break the bow.' Queen Sunaina was relieved.

Sita prayed to Parvati, 'If I have worshiped you with a pure heart, please lighten the bow. I can stay in the forest; take away all my pleasures but please give him strength to lift the bow and break it.'

Parvati was now in a fix. She thought that if she granted Sita her wish, the bow would be broken and Sita would have to lead the life of a mendicant. If she did not grant her wish, she would not get married.

Lakshmana asked the tortoise and Sheshnaag to hold the earth steady, as Rama was all set to break the bow. According to Hindu mythology, the earth is believed to be held in balance by these legendary characters.

Rama bowed to Vishwamitra and started for the podium. He picked up the bow and held it in his left hand. He tried to string the bow by bending it. By the time the assembly could realise what was happening, the bow split into two. The earth trembled with the thunderous sound of the bow breaking. Everyone shut their ears to ward off the sound. Seeing the bow in two pieces, most of the people in the gathering cheered loudly.

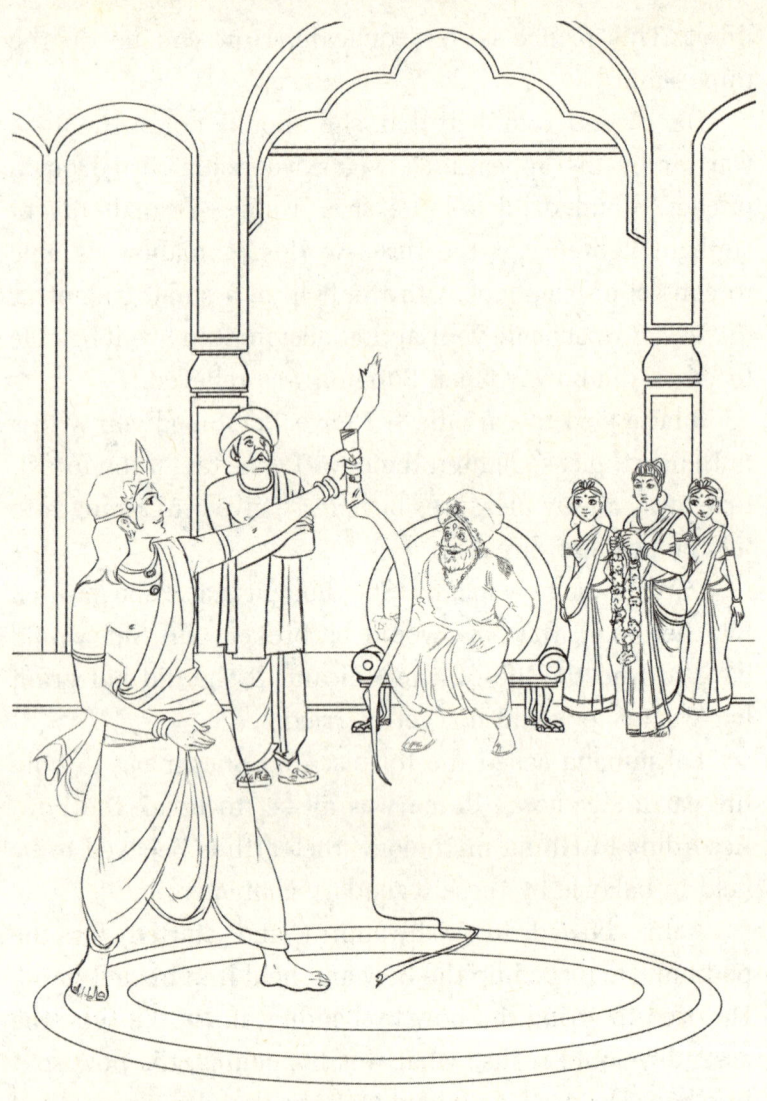

With Satananda's permission, Janaka called for Sita. She held the garland in her hand and walked towards Rama and garlanded him on the podium.

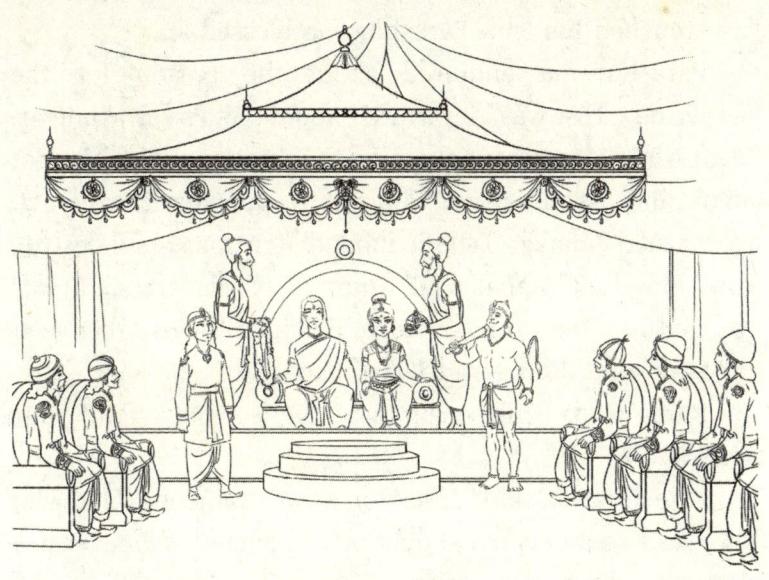

The disgruntled kings drew their swords and said that breaking the bow was immaterial. They vowed to not let Rama take Sita away. And if Janaka chose to intervene, they would defeat him too.

Just then, Parashurama entered the assembly hall. All the kings fell silent out of fear and respect. Parashurama was a great warrior. He was infamous for his short temper. Though he was a Brahmin, he had fought many battles. He had defeated most of the Kshatriyas on earth twenty-one times. He had Kshatriya traits in him just as Vishwamitra had Brahmin traits in him.

They all paid obeisance to him and introduced themselves. Janaka touched his feet. He called Sita and introduced her to Parashurama. Janaka instructed Sita to pay tributes to him. Vishwamitra also came forward and introduced Rama and Lakshmana. Rama and Lakshmana also touched his feet. Parashurama blessed all.

Parashurama enquired about the reason for the gathering. He was informed about Sita's swayamvar. Meanwhile, Parashurama saw the broken bow. He got angry and asked Janaka who was responsible for the act. He warned Janaka, 'Tell me immediately, or I shall destroy your kingdom.' Janaka fell short of words. Sunaina was worried. At that time, a long dialogue ensued between Parashurama, Rama and Lakshmana.

Rama said, 'This seems to be the work of one of your servants.'

Parashurama said, 'A servant serves someone. One who behaves like an enemy should be challenged. Whoever has done this must come forward. He is my enemy, just like Sahastrabahu was at one point of time.'

Lakshmana said, 'In his childhood, I had broken many bows, but you never said anything. Why such special affection for this bow?'

Parashurama said, 'Do you not know this was Lord Shiva's bow? It was not a normal bow.'

Parashurama was known to have wiped out the Kshatriyas from the earth and collected their bows. He had a collection of numerous bows belonging to gods as well. The weight of these bows had started weighing down the earth and Sheshnaag, who is believed to be holding the earth on its hood. So, one day, Mother Earth disguised Sheshnaag as her child and went to Parashurama. She told him that because of her mischievous child, no one was willing to provide them shelter. She asked the rishi if he would take them in. Seeing their plight, Parashurama agreed and said that he would forgive her son's mischief.

One day, when Parashurama had stepped out, Sheshnaag, in the guise of a child, destroyed all the bows except that of Shiva's. When Parashurama returned home, he could not scold him due to the promise. Then, Sheshnaag took his true form and said that this bow of Shiva would be broken by Rama in Treta Yug. Lakshmana reminded Parashurama of this episode.

Lakshmana said, 'The bow was old, so it broke. I will remain silent as one should not show his prowess to gods, Brahmins, devotees and cows. So, even if you attack us, we will not retaliate.'

Parashurama rebuked, 'This boy is insulting me, but I am keeping calm, otherwise I would have killed him and gotten rid of guru *rin* (teacher's debt).'

Lakshmana claimed, 'Who is not familiar with your behaviour? You had cleared your *pitra* and *matra* rin (parent's debt) and *bhatra* rin (brother's debt). Am I supposed to offer my head to you as a guru rin?'

~

A long time ago, Parshurama's father, Rishi Jamdagni, sent his wife, Renuka, to fetch water from the river. Renuka got engrossed in watching a Gandharva and his wife embracing each other, and got delayed. When Jamdagni heard about the reason for the delay, he ordered his sons to slay their mother. All his sons refused. Finally, he ordered Parashurama to slay his mother and brothers. Parashurama obeyed his father. Jamdagni, overwhelmed by his obedience, asked his son to wish for a boon. Parashurama asked that his mother and brothers be brought back to life. This was granted. Thus, by being obedient to his father, he cleared himself from the father's debt, and by saving the lives of his mother and brothers, he cleared himself from their debt as well. Then, he went on a journey of walking around the earth.

Parashurama said, 'Rama, your brother is a sinner.' Rama requested him to forgive his brother.

Lakshmana said, 'Anger is the provenance of all the sins. Anger will not mend the bow. If you permit, I can call a carpenter to repair it.'

Parashurama said, 'I have become calmer now down, otherwise I would not have spared anyone.'

Rama said, 'I am *only* Rama, but you are the great Parashurama. I am no match for you. Please forgive us.'

Then, Parashurama said to Rama, 'The bow in my hand is no less then Shiva's bow. It was given to my grandfather by Lord Vishnu. If you are able to hold this bow, my doubt will be cleared. I will accept you as an incarnation of Vishnu.'

As Parashurama extended his hand with the bow towards Rama, it slid into Rama's hand. Parashurama was amazed! It is said that with the bow, all his powers also went to Rama. Parashurama was also an incarnation of Vishnu with four virtues (*kala*), while Rama was an avatar of Vishnu with twelve virtues. After this incident, Rama became an avatar with sixteen virtues, whereas Parashurama became a mere mortal. He had become very powerful after slaying the Kshatriyas and his act of penance thereafter, which had made him arrogant. To teach him a lesson, Lord Vishnu withdrew all his powers in this manner. Parashurama paid his obeisance to Rama and asked for forgiveness for his harsh words. After this, he left for the forest for atonement.

When all the kings saw Parashurama paying his respects to Rama, they got scared. Now Janaka asked Vishwamitra, 'Even though Sita is married to Rama according to the vow, they need to be accepted by the people as well. What should we do next?'

Vishwamitra suggested sending a messenger to Dasharatha. Janaka agreed and sent the head emissary, Sudaman, to Dasharatha. The messenger reached Ayodhya and gave the letter to the King. Dasharatha was overjoyed. He asked the messenger to narrate the proceedings of the day in detail. Bharata and Shatrughana were very happy to hear the news as well.

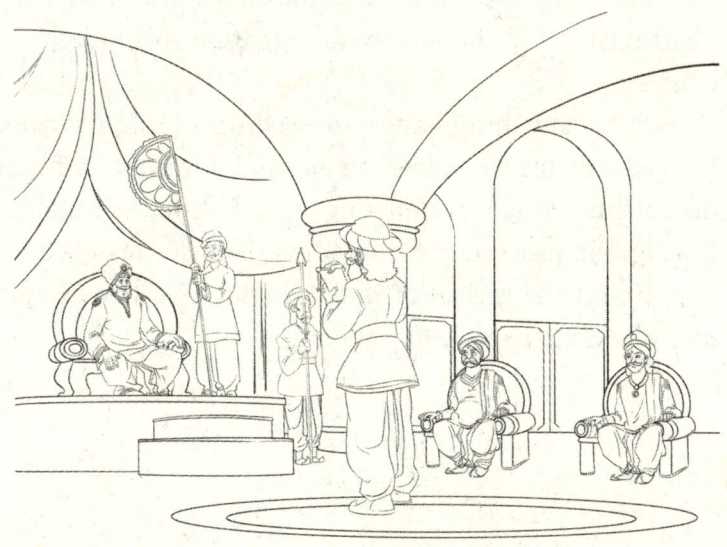

Dasharatha went to his palace and gave the good news to his queens. He asked Bharata to prepare for the wedding procession. Elephants, horses and chariots were decorated, warriors with their bejewelled garments astride them. The procession was launched with the blowing of a conch shell.

The procession reached Mithila after a four-day journey. Janaka came to receive the guests. Rama and Lakshmana were elated on hearing that their father and brothers had arrived. They met each other and paid their respects.

A wedding chart was sent to Janaka. He took it to Satananda. After deciding the programme, marriage rituals were performed. At that time, it was decided that all the four brothers would get married at the same time. Janaka had two daughters. Urmila's wedding was decided with Lakshmana. Janaka had a brother named Kushadhwaja. He had two daughters—Mandvi and Shrutkirti. Mandvi was married to Bharata and Shrutkirti was married to Shatrughana. All the four weddings were solemnized with rituals.

All the four brides were dressed up in *solah shringar* or sixteen bridal adornments and twelve traditional ornaments. After completing the farewell formalities, Dasharatha proceeded for Ayodhya. The queens were very happy with the arrival of their daughters-in-law. A grand *arti* was done to welcome them.

# Journey to the Forest

Days went by, and for once, looking into the mirror, Dasharatha saw a few strands of grey. He thought it was time to announce Rama as the heir to the throne and began arranging for his coronation.

Dasharatha knew that Kaikeyi wanted Bharata to be anointed king. Dasharatha loved Bharata and Kaikeyi, but he wanted to follow the tradition of the family, which said that the eldest son should be the crown prince. Dasharatha started preparations for the ceremony quietly. He sent Bharata to his maternal parents' place, Kekaya Desh. He did not even send an invitation for the ceremony to the family, to avoid any hindrance.

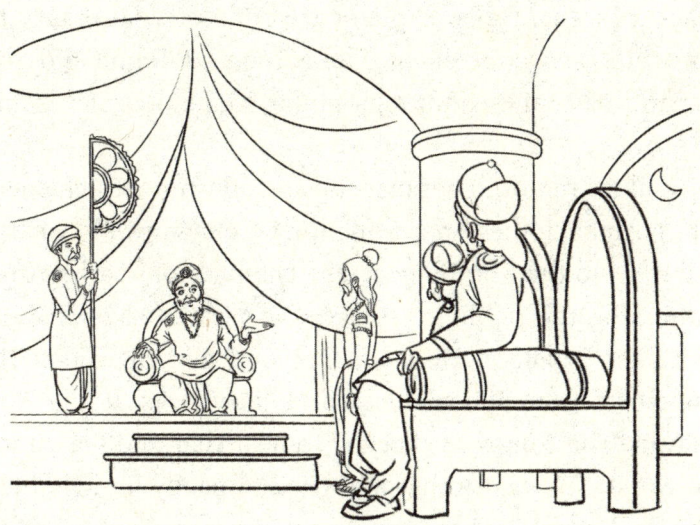

On the eve of the ceremony, Kaikeyi's trusted maid, Manthara, came to know about the event. She hurriedly rushed to inform Kaikeyi. Initially, Kaikeyi could not understand the intricacies of the situation. Manthara helped her understand the outcome of the decision of Rama's coronation.

She had faith in Manthara. She advised Kaikeyi that it was time for her to ask for the two boons to which she was entitled from the King. Manthara said, 'First, you must make the King swear on his Rama's name. Then, demand the boons so that he cannot go back on his promise. He would be ready to die before breaking the promise.'

Manthara also advised that Kaikeyi should ask Dasharatha to first crown Bharata as the crown prince. When this was granted, she should ask for the second boon, else the King might refuse. The second boon was a more devious one—Rama should be exiled for fourteen years. Manthara also explained why it was necessary to send him away for such a long time. If Rama did not go into exile, the conditions might somehow turn in his favour.

Kaikeyi removed her makeup and adornments, changed into normal clothes—not something a queen would wear—and went to the Kop Bhavan (the chamber of wrath). After addressing the public meetings, Dasharatha eagerly went to Kaikeyi's palace. He could not find her anywhere. He found out from the maids that Kaikeyi was at the Kop Bhavan. The King was shocked to hear that and feared for the worst. He went to her and tried to pacify her. He held her hand and asked the reason for her behaviour. Kaikeyi hissed and jerked her hand away. Dasharatha once again asked her the reason.

He said, 'What do you need? I will give whatsoever you demand. Today, I am very happy.'

Kaikeyi said, 'First, swear on Rama that you will provide me whatsoever I demand.'

Dasharatha promised to meet her demands. Kaikeyi said, 'You only enquire but never fulfil the demands. You had promised me two boons but I fear you may refuse that too.'

Dasharatha replied, 'You never asked for them and I too forgot. Anyway, tell me what you desire.'

Kaikeyi said, 'As my first boon, you must announce Bharata as crown prince instead of Rama.'

Dasharatha tried to explain that it is always the eldest son who is made crown prince, but failed to convince her. Dasharatha gave in to her demands and said, 'I shall make Bharata the crown prince. I am sure none of the brothers would mind it, as they love each other very much.'

With a final blow, Kaikeyi asked for the second wish—fourteen years of exile for Rama.

Dasharatha was unable to bear this blow. He staggered and balanced himself by holding on to the furniture close by. He was unable to understand the second wish. Why would she want to send him as away when she loved Rama so much? He requested her to let Rama live in the palace.

Kaikeyi said, 'Either fulfil the boons or accept the blame of breaking your vows.'

Dasharatha was distraught. He pleaded and begged

*Journey to the Forest* 27

Kaikeyi to relent, but Kaikeyi did not change her mind.

Dasharatha did not appear in the court the next day, Sumantra, his minister, went to Dasharatha's palace. Although Sumantra was his finance minister, he was quite close to the King and would also help him with his personal problems. He was more than a friend to the King. He found the King in shambles. It seemed as if he had not slept the whole night. He had been crying through the night and his eyes had turned red. When Sumantra enquired about the matter, the King asked him to fetch Rama for him.

Sumantra rushed to Rama and told him about the King's condition. Rama hurried to Dasharatha and asked him what the matter was.

Dasharatha could not utter a single word and fainted. Kaikeyi entered the chamber and said, 'He cannot tell you anything. I shall tell you. The King had offered me two boons. For the first boon, I asked him to make Bharata the crown prince and as the second boon, I asked him to send you into exile for fourteen years. The King is more attached to you. The thought of being separated from you has put him in this condition. He is torn between love for you and his duties of complying with family traditions. He is in a dilemma and only you can relieve him, by leaving the palace.'

Rama requested Dasharatha to stop grieving and said, 'I will go to the forest. I am fortunate to get a chance to fulfil your wishes.'

When Dasharatha regained consciousness, he embraced Rama. He prayed to Lord Shiva to show him a way to both fulfil the promise and stop Rama from leaving the palace. But all was in vain. Finally, Rama asked for his father's permission to leave for the forest.

Rama went to Kaushalya. He told her everything. Kaushalya too became sad and said that it would have been better if she had remained childless. She also pleaded with Rama not to go.

She said, 'Forget about your father. Stay here in Ayodhya and serve me. Kashyap Rishi attained heaven by serving his mother. Not only a father's wish, a mother's desire also needs to be honoured equally by her son. If you do not obey me, I will kill myself.'

Rama said, 'I cannot dishonour my father.'

Kaushalya argued, 'Okay then. Obey your father. Go to the forest and I will follow you.'

Rama pleaded with his mother to not leave the King and follow him. It was her duty to stay in Ayodhya and serve his father.

At that moment, Sita entered and said that she would accompany Rama to the forest.

On listening to Sita's demand, Kaushalya said that Rama could go if he wanted to, but Sita must stay back. She may stay at Ayodhya or Mithila. She had never seen the hardships of life. She would not be able to live in the forest. Rama also pleaded with Sita but she was adamant on going to the forest. Ultimately, she could convince Rama and Kaushalya and got their permissions.

Lakshmana was furious when he came to know what had happened. He came to Rama and said that he would imprison his father and kill anyone who stopped him. He argued that if a teacher or an elder strayed to the evil path, slaying him would not be a sin. Kaushalya told Rama that he should listen to Lakshmana.

Rama calmed Lakshmana down and explained their family's tradition to him. If they went against the tradition, they would be regarded as the black sheep of their family. Lakshmana then decided to accompany Rama on this journey.

Rama tried to reason with him by asking him to stay back, as one of them needed to be in the Kingdom, given the state of affairs. But Lakshmana was adamant. He touched Rama's feet and begged him not to refuse. Finally, Rama agreed and said that he should go and seek Sumitra Maa's permission.

Lakshmana went to Queen Sumitra and asked for her permission. He was afraid of her refusal.

After hearing the complete story, Sumitra said, 'You go with Rama and Sita to the forest and look after them as if they are your parents. Where there is Rama, there is your Ayodhya.' Lakshmana was pleased to get her permission. When Rama and Lakshmana were ready to leave, Rama told Lakshmana to take Urmila's permission as well.

When Urmila came to know about Rama's exile she said, 'You should fulfil your duties towards your brother. I will do mine as the daughter-in-law here by serving our father and mothers. I will not let them feel your absence.' Lakshmana looked at her with love, and left her chamber filled with pride.

Rama, Lakshmana, Sita and Kaushalya went to see

Dasharatha. Rama informed Dasharatha that Lakshmana and Sita were also going with him.

As a last effort to stop them from going into forest, he said, 'Rama, I am trapped by my vow to honour my promise to Kaikeyi. I advise you to imprison me and take over the throne.'

Rama replied, 'O King! May you rule for a hundred years! I am not greedy for the throne. I will leave now and come back only after fourteen years.'

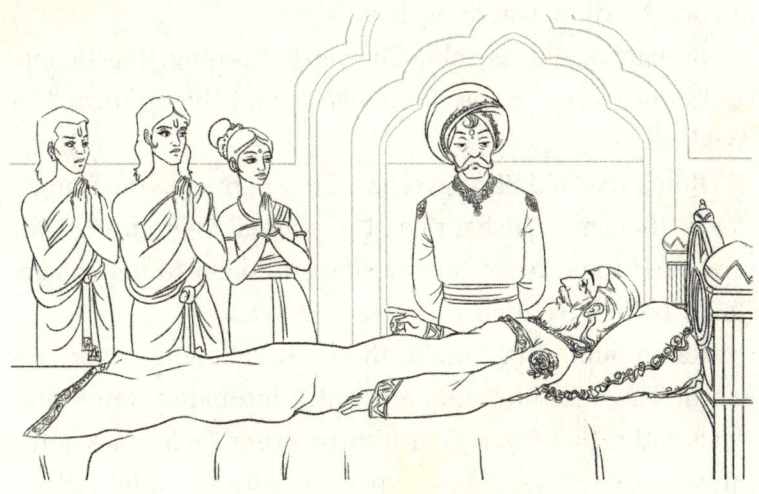

Dasharatha embraced Rama and Lakshmana, weeping all along. He fainted out of grief. When he gained consciousness, he told Sumantra, 'Please take them to the border of the kingdom and stay there for three or four days. Then bring them back. This way, the promise will be fulfilled and Rama would return home. But if the two brothers refuse to come back, make sure you bring Sita back.'

Rama, Lakshmana and Sita sat on the chariot and Sumantra steered them out of the kingdom. Everyone in the kingdom had gathered. They wanted to accompany Rama to the forest. They, along with their people, started the journey towards the forest.

Rama took the first break in his journey at river Tamsa, for a night's halt. At midnight, Rama woke up and spoke to Sumantra. He said, 'Please ready the chariot and let us move out quietly without leaving a trace. I do not want anyone to know where we have gone.'

Sumantra did as told. The next morning, the people could not trace the way Rama went, and they returned to Ayodhya.

Rama reached Shringverpur. They bathed in the Ganga. There they met Nishadraja. He offered them fruits and requested them to let him accompany them to his village. Rama politely refused.

Rama and Sita rested there. Lakshmana stood on guard. The next morning, Sumantra intimated Rama that Dasharatha had instructed him to bring them back after three or four days. Rama explained why he could not go back, and sent Sumantra back to Ayodhya.

Rama, Lakshmana and Sita reached the banks of Ganga and asked the *kewat,* or boatman, to carry them to the other side of the river.

The kewat refused to offer his boat and said, 'This boat is my only source of income. I have heard that the dust of your feet turned a stone into a woman. If it turns my boat into a woman, I will be left with no source of income. But yes, there is a way. Please allow me to wash your feet before stepping into my boat. This way, my boat will remain intact.'

Rama sensed the kewat's wish in the guise of devotion. By collecting the water from Rama's feet, or *charnamrit*, and drinking it, he wished to wash off his sins. Rama smiled and agreed, 'Okay. Do as you wish, but please help us cross the river. Go and fetch the boat.' Such irony! Rama, the incarnation of Vishnu, who helps people cross the devout sea or the Bhav Sagar, was requesting a kewat to take him across the river.

The kewat brought water in a pot and washed Rama's feet. The boatman and his family drank that water. He took Rama, Lakshmana, Sita and Nishadraja across the river. When they disembarked from the boat, Rama looked at Sita and she understood his intention. She took off her ring and gave it to the kewat.

The kewat further said, 'You help people cross the bhav sagar and on earth, I help the people cross the river. Thus, we hail from a similar profession. People of the same profession do not charge each other for their labour. Today, I helped you cross the river. Please help me cross the bhav sagar when I come to you.' Lord Rama smiled and instructed him to go back.

Rama made a Shivling from the sand on the bank of the river and worshiped it. He asked Nishadraja to return, but Nishadraja requested Rama to allow him to accompany him for a while. Rama agreed.

Rama told Lakshmana to be vigilant and prepare to protect Sita, as they were entering the dense forest. He asked Lakshmana to lead and he would follow. Sita was

*Journey to the Forest*

supposed walk between the two of them.

They all reached Rishi Bharadwaj's ashram. After a night's halt, they continued on their journey the next day, with the rishi's disciples. They crossed river Yamuna. Rama asked Nishadraja to now return to his family. They moved ahead towards rishi Valmiki's ashram. Valmiki welcomed them and Rama requested him to help them find an area that was safe to live in. Valmiki advised him to go to Chitrakoot.

Rama, with Lakshmana and Sita, reached Chtirakoot. They surveyed the area. It was beautiful and safe to live in. There was a rivulet nearby. It began at river Mandakini and met the river again, forming a bow. They liked the site and made huts.

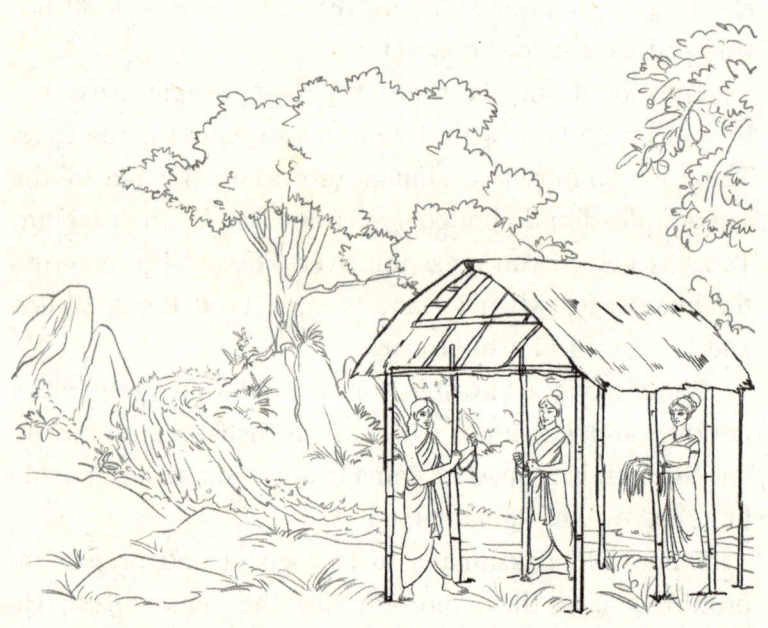

When Sumantra returned to Ayodhya, Dasharatha asked him about Rama, Lakshmana and Sita. Sumantra narrated the whole story and Dasharatha began to lament. He then remembered his curse and told Kaushalya about it.

He said, 'While hunting in the forest in Ayodhya, I was waiting near a river hoping to find my kill. I heard a sound and shot a Shabd Bhed Baan in its direction. This arrow could detect sound and follow it. When I reached the spot, I was shocked to see a boy struck by the arrow crying in pain. This boy was Shravan Kumar, who had come to the river to fetch water for his blind parents. He had been carrying them on his shoulders with the help of a sling. The boy requested me to take the pitcher of water to his parents. His parents cursed me for what had happened. They said, "You will die of grief caused by the separation from your son in your old age".'

Dasharatha did not pay heed to their words as he did not have a son then. He died lamenting the separation from his sons.

Vasishtha placed the King's body in a boat and poured oil over it. He sent a messenger to fetch Bharata and Shatrughana from Kekaya Desh.

Bharata was constantly feeling restless but could not guess the reason. After a journey of seven days, Bharata reached Ayodhya and was welcomed by Kaikeyi.

Bharata asked his mother, 'Why is the city so quiet? Where are father and my brothers?'

Kaikeyi informed him about his father's demise. Bharata was shocked to hear this. Then he asked where

*Journey to the Forest*

Rama Bhaiya and the rest were. Kaikeyi told him the whole story. Bharata got furious and rebuked his mother. At that time, Manthara entered the room. Shatrughana flew into a violent rage and assaulted her. Bharata intervened and said that women should be respected at all times.

Vasishtha asked Bharata to perform his father's last rites. Then, the sage asked Bharata to take over as king. Bharata said, 'I will agree to everything you propose, but first, I want to meet Bhaiya Rama.' Everyone thought this was the right thing to do.

Bharata called his trusted guards and instructed them to look after Ayodhya, and the next day, Bharata, along with the three mothers, his ministers and the army, left for the forest to meet Rama.

When Nishadraja saw them, he thought their intentions were wrong and ordered all boatmen to immerse their boats and oars into the water. As a result, no one could cross the river. The elders in the village suggested to first check why they were here, and then take appropriate action. On learning that Bharata's intentions were good, Nishadraja took him to Rama.

On seeing Bharata with an army, Lakshmana got furious. He was ready to attack him when Rama calmed him down.

Everyone reached Chitrakoot and met Rama. They were informed about Dasharatha's death and that Vasishtha had performed the last rites. The same day, Janaka also reached Chitrakoot.

The next day, everyone tried to convince Rama to return to Ayodhya. Rama explained that it would not be the right thing to do and that he must stay there and follow his father's instructions. Bharata should look after Ayodhya.

Bharata said that he would need some sort of support which would help him get through fourteen years. Rama gave him his *khadau*, or wooden slippers. Bharata respectfully kept them on his head.

Bharata stayed there for a week and went back to Ayodhya with the entire retinue.

On reaching Ayodhya, Bharata called his ministers and trusted staff. He explained to them the working of the State. He deputed Shatrughana to the service of the mothers. He placed Rama's khadau on the throne as an embodiment of his brother and, dressed as a hermit, he stayed at Nandigram.

Meanwhile, at Chitrakoot, Rama, Lakshmana and Sita were getting used to the forest life and the days were passing by peacefully. One day, Rama was sitting outside the cottage and adorning Sita with jewellery made of flowers. Lord Indra's son Jayant, disguised as a crow, flew into the ashram. He pecked at Sita's feet and flew away. Her feet started bleeding. Rama became angry and picked up a straw and threw it at the crow. The straw, fortified by Rama's words, followed the crow and brought it down. The crow took its real form and Jayant hid behind his father, Lord Indra.

Indra knew Rama's might and said, 'I cannot save you.' Just like the fear of Sudarshan Chakra had once driven Sage Durvasa helter-skelter, Jayant too fled for his life between the three worlds, but no one offered him refuge. No one wanted to associate with an enemy of Rama. Just then, Sage Narad came and advised him to seek refuge from Rama himself. Jayant rushed helplessly to Rama in tears.

Rama said, 'It is impossible to stop the weapon but I will reduce its harmful effect. It will not kill you, but you shall be blind in one eye.'

After spending some time in Chitrakoot, Rama started for the Sage Atri's ashram. Sita met sage Atri's wife Ansuiya. Sita touched her feet. She gifted Sita divine clothes which would always remain fresh and clean. She gave her a divine necklace as well. She also taught her the characteristics of a good wife. After meeting Sage Atri, Rama moved on.

The trio then reached Sage Sharbhang's Ashram. They moved ahead, and on their way, Rama noticed a heap of bones. Rama enquired what it was. The sages accompanying him said that they were the bones of sages killed by demons. Rama was upset and vowed that he would extinguish all demons from earth.

Rama met Suteekshan. He was Sage Agastya's disciple. Once, Agastya gave him a small *sinhasan,* or throne, with a stone on it. The smooth, round and black stone symbolized Vishnu and was called Shaligram. The sage instructed him to take care of it. Some time later, Suteekshan was passing through a forest and crossed a jamun (blackberry) tree. He wanted to eat the fruit. He looked around wondering how to pluck it. When he could not find a stone or stick, he hurled the Shaligram towards the bunch of fruits on the tree. After eating the Jamun, he remembered about the shaligram. He started searching for it. When he could not find it, he picked up a jamun fruit and placed it on the sinhasan in lieu of Shaligram. The next morning, Sage Agastaya during his prayer held the blueberry (taking it to be Shaligram) and washed it with water, rubbing it mildly. The fruit's skin came off and so did its flesh. Only the seed remained in his hand. The sage became furious and snapped at Suteekshan. Suteekshan replied,

> 'Puni puni chandan puni puni pani!
> Gal gaya thakur hum ka jani!'

Which means: 'You have been giving it a bath daily and smearing sandalwood paste on it. It seems that Thakur (Lord Vishnu) has melted away due to the excess water. How do I know what happened?' In a fit of rage, the sage shut him away from the Lord. It was the same Suteekshan whom Rama met in the forest. Suteekshan thought, since he was not a good devotee or follower of rituals, Rama may not like meeting him, but Rama greeted him very affectionately. He even decided to meet Sage Agastaya.

Since Rama was going to meet Agastya, Suteekshan also decided to accompany him. He said, 'I too have not met the sage for a very long time. Please allow me to accompany you.'

Rama agreed. They all went to the Sage's Ashram.

When they reached the ashram, Suteekshan said in a loud voice, 'See guru ji (teacher), whom I have brought along. Look, it's the Lord.'

The Sage rushed out from the cottage with tears in eyes. Rama and Lakshmana touched his feet. The Sage pulled them into a tight embrace. He also blessed Suteekshan and said, 'I had reprimanded and ordered you to bring back the

Shaligram. But you have brought the Lord himself.'

Rama, Lakshmana and Sita stayed at the Agastaya Ashram for some time. Under the guidance of the rishi, Rama could fulfil his vow, and killed 14,000 demons. Agastaya gave him a bow named Aeind, a quiver with an inexhaustible supply of arrows, and a sword. Agastaya suggested that Rama should reside in Panchwati, the area between Shaval and Vindhyachal hills. Once, it was under the rule of King Dand. The king had assaulted Saga Shukracharya's daughter. The sage cursed him, and his kingdom turned into a forest. Since then, the kingdom was known as Dandkaranya. Sages and rishis, finding it quite and calm, used it for their worship. Inhabited by holy people seeking peace, this area was soon renamed to Jansthan.

Rama moved on and met Jatayu, the Vulture King, near Panchwati. Rama set up his cottage near river Godavari and settled down. Gradually, their friendship grew. The area was an example of scenic beauty. It was suitable in case a war ensued. On one side, there was river Godavari and on the other were small hillocks. The cottage was located at a height which offered good visibility. In case of an attack, one could hide behind a hillock and fight.

# The Abduction of Sita

Brahma had a human son named Rishi Pulastya. Pulastya had a son named Rishi Vishrava. Vishrava was married to Devangana. He was a firm believer of pure thoughts, deeds and actions. Kuber, also known as Vaisravana, was his son. Pleased by his charity and penance, Lord Brahma anointed Kuber as his fourth *lokpal*, or the protector of the universe, and gifted him a Pushpak Viman, which could be navigated as per the rider's wishes.

Kuber got a boon from Lord Brahma. He went to his father and said, 'I have earned the blessings of Lord Brahma. Now, tell me where I should settle down.'

Vishrava told him that the mid-hillocks of Trikut *Parwat,* or hill, are vast and green. On its peak, was a beautiful city named Lankapuri which had been constructed by Vishwakarma. He advised him to go and settle there.

Earlier, some rakshasas were residing in Lankapuri. Lord Vishnu had slayed them and the surviving rakshasas were forced to go to the netherworld. Among these was a rakshas named Sumali. He was very ambitious. He wanted to recapture Lankapuri, but could not find a single rakshas who had the courage and determination to help him fulfil his dream.

He wanted a son who could consolidate and direct the strength of the rakshasas into a united fighting force. As Kuber was controlling Lanka, it was logical to have someone from the same lineage to cement his empowerment.

In tune with this thought, he called his daughter Kaikesi and coaxed her into marring Vishrava. Kaikesi went to Vishrava and told him that upon her father's coaxing, she had come to marry the Sage and beget a son.

The Sage replied that since she had approached him in the evening, which is dark, their children would have bad temperaments. Kaikesi said that since they would be his sons too, they would definitely inherit his intelligence and charitable nature. The Sage said that one of her children would be a great religious and pious man.

Kaikesi had three sons and one daughter with the Sage. The eldest was Ravana, the second Kumbhkarana, third was their daughter Shurpanakha and the pious one, Vibhishana, was the fourth child. Ravana had traits of both his parents—father, a sage, and mother, a demon—infused into his personality. He was a great worshiper of Lord Shiva. He was brave, intelligent, a music lover, a good politician, a good ruler and a great pandit, but he was a stubborn, arrogant and ambitious person. Kumbhkarana was huge and strong. Vibhishana was a devotee of Vishnu.

All the three brothers went and worshiped at Sage Gokarana's Ashram. Ravana severed his nine heads and when he was about to sever the tenth, Lord Brahma appeared to grant him his desired boon. Lord Brahma regrew all his nine heads and granted him the ability to appear in any form he wished. Then, he asked Ravana if there was anything else that he desired, as Lord Brahma was very pleased with him. Ravana asked for immortality, to which Brahma said that this was a wish that he could not grant. Brahma told him to ask for anything else. Ravana asked Brahmaji to provide him with complete protection or immunity against serpents, garuda, yakshs, demons and demigods—he should be unassailable to any attack from them. His arrogance led him to not consider humans or animals harmful. Lord Brahma immediately said, 'So be it.'

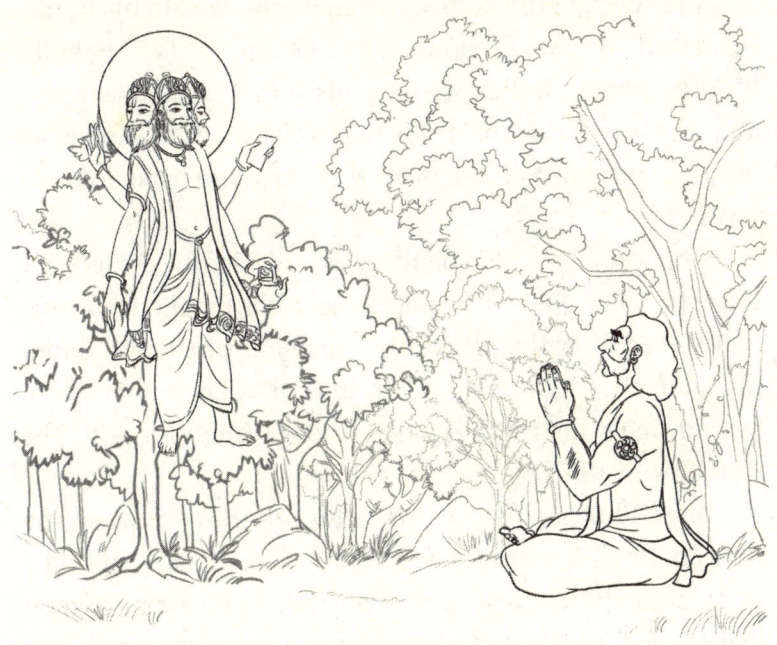

Then, Brahma went to Kumbhkarana and asked about his wish. He was huge and so was his diet, because of which the gods feared that he might gobble up all the creatures on earth to satisfy his hunger. They requested Goddess Saraswati to intervene. She could help in altering Kumbhakarana's mind.

Kumbhkarana was fascinated with the *Indraasan*, Lord Indra's throne. He wanted to ask for it, but Saraswati changed his mind and he asked for the Nidraasan, or the throne of the sleep god. Brahmaji agreed and said, 'So be it.'

Finally, Brahmaji asked Vibhishana his desire. Vibhishana said that he only wanted his blessings. Brahmaji said, 'So be it, and along with it, you get immortality.'

After getting the boons, Ravana went back to his home. He asked for the Kingdom of Lankapuri from his elder brother Kuber. Kuber went to his father, Sage Vishrava, and conveyed Ravana's wish. His father told Kuber to be generous and hand over the Kingdom of Lanka to Ravana.

Shurpanakha's husband was accidently killed by Ravana. Since then, she emotionally blackmailed Ravana. She looked after the picket of Janasthan, which was under the control of Lanka, with her cousins Khar and Dushan. On Ravana's instructions, they caused hindrances in the worships of the sages.

Once, Shurpanakha was on a tour of the area when she noticed Rama's cottage—Parnakuti. Out of curiosity, she went near the cottage. She was smitten by Rama's good looks. She transformed herself into a beautiful woman and approached him.

She said, 'There is no man as handsome as you on the earth, and there is no lady who can match my beauty. So, I want to marry you.'

Rama said, 'I am already married and have taken a vow to be loyal to my wife. Here is my younger brother.'

Then, Shurpanakha approached Lakshmana who reacted in a similar manner when she tried to express her love to him.

Lakshmana turned her away and said, 'Rama is the King of Ayodhya and I am his servant. I cannot provide you the luxury that he can. Therefore, I advise you to go back to him.'

Shurpanakha again went back to Rama. In this way, she went back and forth between Rama and Lakshmana and became an object of jest for the two brothers. They started making fun of her.

Shurpanakha realised that she was being rejected by them due to Sita. Then, she transformed herself back to her real form and yelled at Rama, 'You are rejecting me for Sita. You will have no choice if I kill her.'

And she rushed to attack Sita. Sita got scared and did not know how to react. Rama came in front of Sita and ordered Lakshmana to punish Shurpanakha. Lakshmana cut off her nose and ears. She howled in pain.

Shurpanakha returned to the camp and narrated the whole story to her cousin Khar and Dushan. She instigated them to challenge Rama.

Shurpanakha attacked Rama with fourteen demons but he killed all of them. Shurpanakha went back to the camp and came back with Khar and Dushan and with their armies.

Rama instructed Lakshmana to go and hide with Sita in the hills. Lakshmana was reluctant, but on Rama's insistence, took her away. Rama slew all the demons.

Then, Shurpanakha rushed to Ravana and narrated the

whole story and provoked him to avenge her humiliation. She also told him that Khar, Dushan and Trishira had been killed in this battle.

She told Ravana about Sita's beauty and enticed him to abduct and wed her. Shurpanakha suggested to Ravana that he should defeat Rama and make him her servant. She reminded Ravana that he had killed her husband, and now it was time to pay her back.

Ravana thought that if Rama was able to kill Khar and Dushan, who were as powerful as Ravana, then he was definitely a powerful warrior. Meanwhile, one of his informants named Prahast, came to him and narrated the entire story again. Ravana was enraged and thought of fighting Rama. Instead, Prahast suggested that he should abduct Sita, as this way it would be easier to defeat Rama. The pangs of separation from Sita will be too much for Rama to bear. That alone would kill him. Ravana found this plan worthy and fool proof.

Now, to materialise his plan he went to Marich, son of Tadaka. This was the same Marich whom Rama had struck with an arrow, which flung him far away, during the fight with Tadaka. Ravana disclosed his plan. Marich tried to reason with him and asked, 'Which fool has advised you this plan? He certainly is your enemy. Rama is very powerful. I was struck by his arrow. It is impossible to win against him in battle. Let him stay in the forest with his wife and you enjoy your life in your palace with your women.'

Ravana replied, 'Either you agree with me and join me in my plan, or I will kill you.'

Marich thought it would be foolish to challenge him since he was armed, knowledgeable, wealthy and a Brahmin. He further thought that if he had to die, then why not die by the hands of Rama. He agreed to Ravana's plan.

Ravana explained to him his strategy. He said, 'You will assume the form of a golden deer and distract Rama and Lakshmana. In the meantime, I will kidnap Sita.'

As per the plan, Marich came near Parnakuti disguised as a golden deer. When Sita saw the deer she told Rama, 'Lord, this deer is very beautiful. Please catch it for me.'

Rama said, 'It seems to be a trick. Have you ever seen a golden deer?'

Sita was adamant and requested Rama to catch it. To please her, Rama picked up his bow and arrow. Before leaving the place, he instructed Lakshmana, 'There are demons and wild animals in the forest. Be vigilant and protect Sita. I shall return after hunting the deer.'

The deer ran deeper into the forest with Rama close on its heels. Ultimately, Rama aimed and shot the deer. Marich cried out loudly in Rama's voice 'Oh Lakshmana!' and in his heart he uttered the name of Lord Rama. Marich appeared in his real form and died. After killing Marich, Rama hurried back to the cottage. He feared for Sita's safety after realising this could have been a trap.

Meanwhile, when Sita heard someone cry 'Lakshmana', she thought that Rama was in trouble.

She commanded, 'Lakshmana, it appears your brother is in trouble. Go and help him.'

Lakshmana said, 'Mother, it is impossible that brother

could be in any kind of trouble. He has instructed me not to leave you alone. I cannot disobey him.' Eventually he reluctantly agreed to do as Sita asked.

Before leaving the cottage, he drew a line around it called the Lakshmana Rekha, for her protection. He requested Sita not to cross it. Even today, this line is synonymous with 'staying within limits'. Lakshmana set off with his bow and arrow in the direction of the cry.

Meanwhile, Ravana, in the guise of a hermit, came to the cottage begging for *bhiksha* or alms. He sensed danger when he tried to cross the Lakshmana Rekha. He called out for alms. Sita reached out to the mendicant and tried to give him alms from within the line as advised by Lakshmana.

Ravana said, 'I do not want to be given alms like a beggar. Take it back or come out and hand it over with respect.'

He began to move away. Sita was perplexed. She knew that turning a hermit away without alms was a sin. So, she stepped out of the boundary. Immediately, Ravana grabbed her, put her on his chariot and flew away.

Sita began to cry, 'O Master, O Lakshmana, please save me.' Hearing her cries for help, the Vulture King Jatayu, who lived nearby, tried to stop Ravana. Ravana caught hold of Jatayu's hair and flung him to the ground. But he did not give up. Jatayu wounded Ravana by continuously pecking him. Ravana cut off Jatayu's wings and he fell to the ground moaning and groaning with pain. Ravana again grabbed Sita and flew off in his chariot.

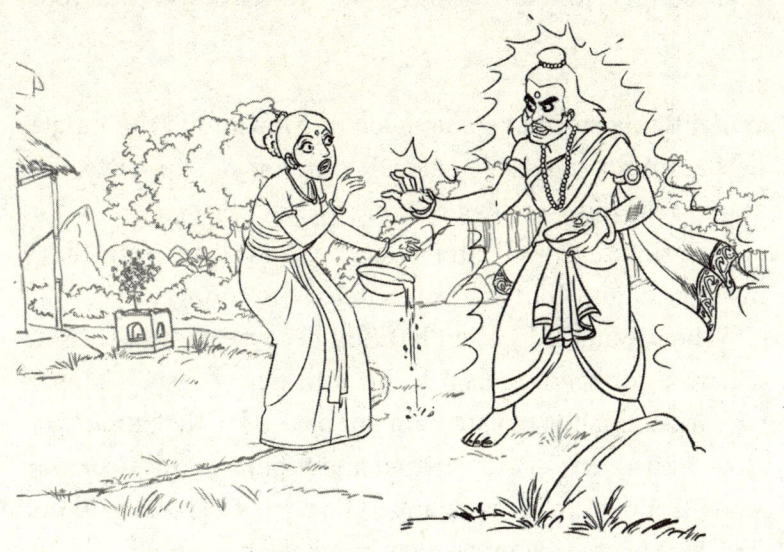

Sita dropped her jewellery one by one along the way, leaving a trail for Rama and hoping that they would lead him to her. On the way, she saw a bunch of monkeys on a hillock. She bundled up the rest of the jewellery in a cloth and dropped it near them. Ravana drove off to Lankapuri.

Ravana had made all arrangements for Sita at the Ashok Vatika. Sita was so sad that she refused to have even a morsel of food.

Elsewhere, Lord Brahma told Lord Indra, 'Sita is in Lanka, beyond the sea. How and when will Rama come to know her whereabouts? She has been refusing food too. How long can she stay alive without food? If she dies before Rama locates her, our entire mission will fail. Take this kheer with you and ensure that Sita eats it. She will then be able to live without food.' Indra did as was told.

⁂

When Rama saw Lakshmana looking for him in the jungle, he became furious. He said, 'I told you not to leave Sita alone. Why did you disobey me?'

Lakshmana told him that he had come on Sita's insistence, and that she was safe in the cottage.

Then Rama said, 'You left Sita because she was upset? Did you not see a reason to be with her yourself? This is very irresponsible of you. I am not pleased with your action. Now let us hurry. I am worried about Sita, as this deer was actually a demon. This seems to be a trick.' They could not find Sita anywhere when they reached the cottage.

Rama was distraught and began to lament. He went to every flower and tree and asked about Sita. Lakshmana was unable to bear seeing his brother in this condition.

While desperately looking for any evidence that he could chance upon, Rama came across the wounded Jatayu. Rama caressed his head gently. Jatayu was relieved of his pain. He told Rama that Ravana had carried Sita away. He said, 'I tried to stop Ravana but failed. I was only waiting to intimate you about Sita. Now I can die in peace.'

Jatayu died. Rama was deeply saddened by his death. Rama cremated him and after performing his last rites, along with Lakshmana, he started for Rishi Matang's Ashram.

All of a sudden, a storm broke out and a huge demon came growling and snarling at them. He was massive and had no head or neck. His body had only a torso with very long arms. There was a mouth and a red eye on his stomach. Due to his appearance, he had been named Kabandh, which literally means 'ugly giant'. He held Rama and Lakshmana in his hands and tried to gobble them. But the brothers cut off his arms. The fight ended and they introduced themselves to Kabandh.

Kabandh narrated his story to them. He said, 'I was a handsome Gandharva (a celestial musician), named Vishvavasu, and spent my time scaring sages. Sage Sthulshira cursed me to remain in the hideous form that I took to scare him. I worshiped Lord Brahma and was granted immortality. Blessed with the boon, I became arrogant and attacked Lord Indra. During the fight, Indra struck me with a mace on my head. With one blow, he drove my head and legs into my torso. When I begged for his forgiveness, he gave me two long arms and a mouth on my belly. When I apologized and requested him to relinquish me of the curse, he said that Rama and Lakshmana will sever my hands and cremate me. Only then will I return to my original form.'

Rama also narrated his story to Kabandh. In the end, he told him that a demon had abducted his wife. Rama said, 'I know the name of that demon but not how he looks or where he lives. I will cremate you but if you know anything about Ravana, please tell me.'

Kabandh said, 'When you cremate me, my divine powers will come back. Then, I will tell you the whereabouts of the person who might be able to help you.'

As soon as Rama and Lakshmana cremated him, he came out of the fire in the form of a divine being.

He said, 'In this world there are six policies, abiding

which a king can fulfil his desires. They are: Sandhi (co-operation), Vigrah (war and division), Yaan (movement), Aasan (seat of power), Dwairthnhav (hypocrisy/diplomacy) and Samashraya (equality).'

He further said, 'One should treat people equally. This also includes being friends with those who live under similar circumstances. This is the law of empathy. Birds of the same feathers flock together.'

He said, 'King Rikshraja had two sons, Vali and Sugriva. Sugriva is also considered to be the son of the Sun God. He has the knowledge of each and every demon on earth. He shall find Sita wherever she may be. Sugriva was forced to leave his kingdom and his wife was also taken away. He will understand your problem and empathise with you. He stays on Rishimukh Hill, which stretches up to Pampa Lake, with his four loyal ape friends. You should go and meet him. He is also in search of a friend like you.'

After this, Rama and Lakshmana set out on their journey. On their way, they came across the hermitage of Shabri. She offered her salutations to Rama and Lakshmana. She offered them fruits and other eatables. She first tasted the berries herself and then offered them the sweet ones only. She put the sour ones aside. Rama took one berry at a time and ate them, relishing their taste. Lakshmana did not like her offering the tasted berries. He wondered why Rama was having these half-eaten berries. He dared not object to Rama, but he did not eat the berries himself. He quietly hurled them away. It is believed that these berries fell over Dronagiri Parvat, where the life-saving herb Sanjeevani

Booti grew. The same herb was given to Lakshmana to save his life, when he was struck by the very powerful weapon Shakti by Meghnad, Ravana's son.

Rama asked Shabri that if she had any news of Sita. Shabri advised them to go to Rishimuk Parvat near Pampa Lake. She said that there he would find the whereabouts of Sita.

Lord Rama reached Pampa Lake. There were hermitages there. The forest was filled with fruit-bearing trees. He took a bath there. All the gods came to meet him. When all of them left, Narad came to pay Rama a visit.

Narad was once attracted to a princess and wanted to marry her. He went to Vishnu and prayed for a face resembling Hari. Narad did not know 'Hari' also meant a monkey. During the swayamvar, the princess chose Vishnu instead of Narad and everyone mocked and laughed at him. He cursed Vishnu that he would lose his beloved and endure the pains of separation. In order to get her back, he would have to befriend monkeys.

After exchanging pleasantries, Narad said, 'When I was enamoured with your magical creation, you did not let me marry the woman and now you are upset about being separated from your wife. Now I feel bad that you have been separated from your wife because of my curse. But the monkeys will help you now. You have reached the right place.'

# The Slaying of Vali

Rama led the way and reached the hillock of Rishimukh, where Sugriva was camping with his ministers. When Sugriva saw them approaching, he instructed Hanuman to go and check who these two strong and handsome men were. If they had been sent by Vali, they will have to run for their lives. Sugriva advised Hanuman to disguise himself as a Brahmin.

As advised, Hanuman approached Rama and Lakshmana and asked them who they were and the purpose of their visit.

Rama said, 'We are the sons of Dasharatha and have come to the forest to abide by our father's instructions. My wife has been abducted by a demon, and we are searching for her. Now please tell us, who are you?'

After hearing this, Hanuman recognized them. He fell on Rama's feet and asked for his forgiveness for failing to recognize them instantly. He further asked, 'But, my Lord, how come you did not recognize me?'

Hanuman transformed himself into his original form. Rama embraced him and said, 'Please do not get me wrong. You are dearer to me than Lakshmana. Everyone knows that I treat everyone equally, but the truth is that I have extra affection for devotees like you.'

Hanuman then said, 'The King of Monkeys, Sugriva, stays on this hill. He is your servant now. But he is scared.

Please rid him of his fears and become his friend. He could send hundreds of monkeys in all directions to look for Mother Sita.'

Hanuman carried both the brothers on his shoulders and took them to Sugriva. Sugriva was very pleased to see the two brothers, and he embraced Rama with affection. Hanuman narrated Rama's story to Sugriva and Sugriva's to Rama and they pledged their friendship for one another, keeping fire as a witness.

After becoming friends, Sugriva told Rama, 'Lord, you need not worry. We shall find Janakiji. Some time back, when I was sitting here, I saw Janakiji being carried away, in a Pushpak Vimaan. We all noticed that she was crying out for help. When she saw us she threw a bundle of her jewellery down near us.'

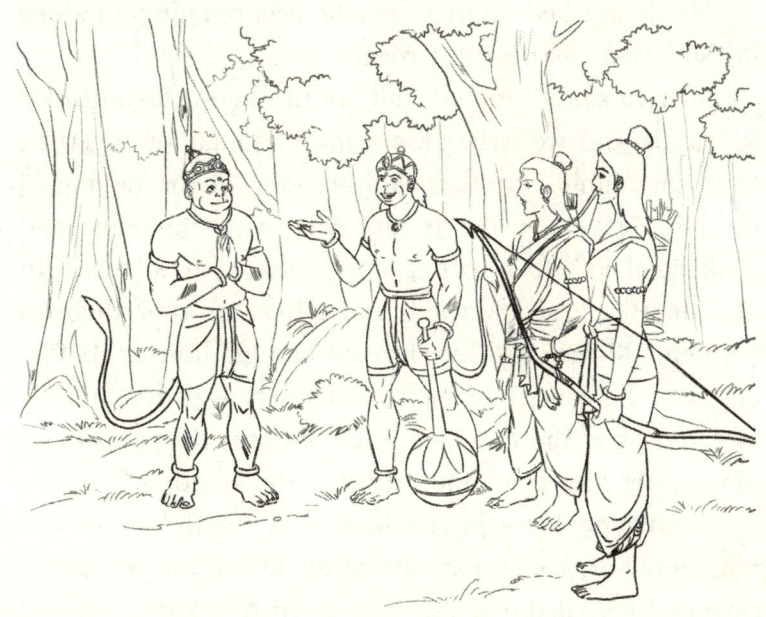

*The Slaying of Vali* 55

Rama asked Sugriva to show him the jewellery. Sugriva immediately fetched the bundle.

Rama, on seeing the jewellery, recognized them and told Lakshmana, 'These are Sita's jewellery, her ear tops, armlets and anklets.'

Lakshmana replied that he did not recognize the ear tops or armlets as he always spoke to Sita with his eyes cast down, but he did recognize her anklets. Rama clung to the jewellery and pondered apprehensively. He was worried and anxious.

Sugriva tried to pacify him and said, 'Lord, please don't worry. I will try my best to look for Janakiji and will definitely find her.'

Rama replied, 'You have treated me as a true friend and your assurance has put me at ease.'

He then asked Sugriva why he was roaming all alone in the forest, bereft of his royalty.

Sugriva said, 'Me and Vali are brothers. Our father is Rikshraja and we were all staying very happily together. Once Dundubhi's brother, Mayavi—son of the demon of illusion, Mayevi—came to our village at midnight and challenged Vali to a battle. Mayavi ran away at the sight of Vali. He chased Mayavi, and I too ran after them to help Vali. Mayavi entered the cave and hid himself. Before entering the cave, Vali instructed me to wait for him for fifteen days at the entrance. If he did not come out, I was to consider him dead and return to the kingdom.'

Sugriva further said, 'I waited for a month but Vali did not come out. I saw a stream of blood coming out of the cave and feared the worst. I assumed that Vali had been killed and now the demon would come out and kill me too. So I ran back to the kingdom but before leaving, I sealed the mouth of the cave with a large boulder. The ministers pressurized me to become king, as the kingdom without a king is open to all kinds of threats. Vali returned after a few days after killing Mayavi. Seeing me on the throne, he thought I had deceived him. He punished and tortured me like I was an enemy and took away all my wealth and even my wife. I was scared for my life, and since, then have been hiding and running from one place to another. Then, I came to Rishimukh Hill and have been staying here ever since because this is the only place where Vali would never come. He has been cursed by Sage Matang that if he ever ventures into Rishimukh Hill, he will lose his life.'

After listening to the whole story, Rama told Sugriva, 'Vali can be killed with a single arrow.'

Sugriva contested, 'Vali is too powerful and mighty. He also has a boon that half of the strength of his opponent would get transferred to him the moment the contender looks into his eyes. So, he would always be a winner. He has also defeated Ravana.'

He showed Rama the heap of Dundubhi's bones under the tree, which Vali had collected after killing him. Rama demolished the heap with a slight nudge. Sugriva was very happy and was convinced of Rama's strength.

He told Rama, 'I am assured that you can slay Vali. I shall forgo all happiness, bliss, wealth, family and fame and shall become your servant forever. Now, I will consider Vali as my greatest well-wisher, for it is because of him that I have met you.'

Rama and Sugriva walked together. Rama suggested that Sugriva should challenge Vali to a duel. He would attack him from a hidden place and kill him.

They approached the palace and Sugriva, backed by Rama, roared loudly and challenged Vali to a duel. Hearing his challenge, Vali began to walk out of the palace, but was stopped by his wife Tara. She told him that the two brothers accompanying Sugriva were the sons of King Dasharatha, and they had the courage and power to take on death itself. Tara could see the future. Vali did not pay any heed to his wife's warnings. He came out and attacked Sugriva. He struck a mighty blow and Sugriva was thrown into the distance.

Scared, Sugriva ran back to Rama and said, 'Lord, I told you, he is not my brother. He is my *Kaal* (doom).'

Rama said, 'You brothers are so alike that I could not make out which one is Vali. Thus, I could not shoot him.'

Rama gently caressed Sugriva, and all his pain vanished. He then gave Sugriva a garland so that he could differentiate between the two brothers. Sugriva returned to the duel.

Rama hid behind a tree. Sugriva and Vali engaged in a fierce battle. Sugriva fought valiantly but Vali was too powerful for him. Then, Rama shot an arrow that struck Vali straight in the heart.

Struck by Rama's arrow, Vali fell on the ground. Rama appeared in front of him when he was breathing his last.

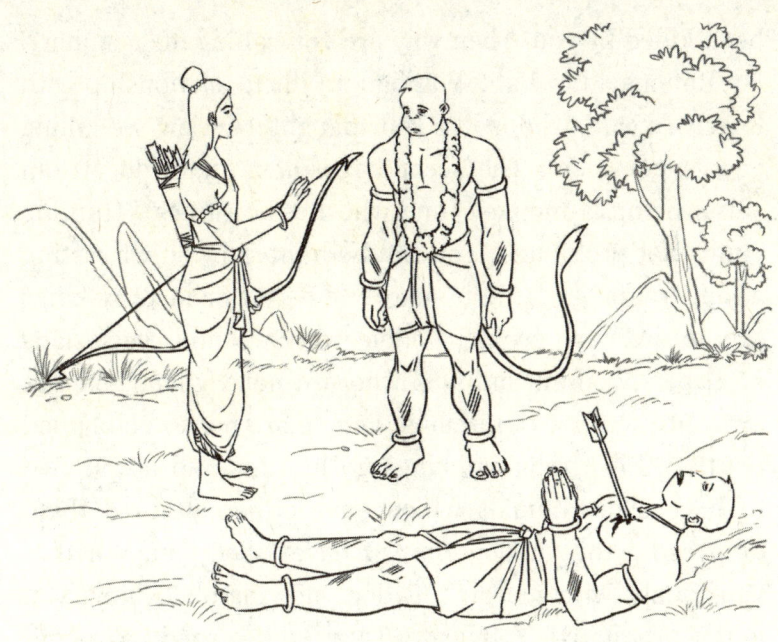

Vali said to Rama, 'Lord, you have been incarnated to establish faith and religion, but you have killed me with deceit. It seems that I am your enemy and Sugriva is your ally, why? Why, my Lord, did you kill me in this manner?'

Rama said, 'A younger brother's wife, a sister, a daughter-in-law and a daughter are all alike. Anyone who casts an evil eye on them needs to be killed. It is not at all unethical to kill such a person. This is Bharata's kingdom and I represent the King. I am bound to uphold faith and religion and destroy anything that contradicts them. Helping anyone who has always upheld faith and religion is my prime duty and it is also considered to be a religious duty.'

Vali said, 'I am going to your abode (heaven), as I have

been killed by you. Then why are you calling me a sinner?'

Rama said to Vali, 'You had an illicit relationship with Sugriva's wife, who is like your daughter-in-law. So killing you is not a sin. The second reason is that you are an aerial being, a monkey (one who lives on trees). Hunting you is not prohibited. You can he hunted by either casting a net, trapping you in a snare, by deceit or tact, by kings or the ordinary people. People who are non-vegetarians or Kshatriya, hunt animals who are not vigilant and run away at the sight of humans. People are not to be blamed for that. Even religious kings go hunting and are known to have slain animals which have either attacked them or posed a threat. Therefore, I have killed you. Whether you fought with me or not, does not matter. Killing you is not prohibited. Your wife, Tara, had warned you about me. But you turned a deaf ear to her advice and accepted Sugriva's challenge. You fought with him and tried to kill him. Despite everything, if you want, I can grant you life.'

Vali, with folded hands, said, 'Lord, after being killed by you, I am ensured a place in heaven. Why should I ask for another life? But I have a request. Please take my son, Angad, under your protection. I have nothing to worry about except for the betterment of my son. Please accept him and Sugriva, and give them the same affection and love that you have for Bharata and Lakshmana. Please do not exploit or ill-treat my wife Tara or my brother Sugriva due to my sins.'

Vali had a necklace with very special powers. He gave the same to Sugriva and told him to put it on immediately, because once he died, its powers would be gone if not worn immediately. Sugriva took his advice, and wore the necklace.

Vali's wife came wailing down from the palace. Rama calmed her. He advised Sugriva to arrange for a proper cremation, with all rites and rituals, for Vali. He then advised Lakshmana to go and arrange for the coronation of Sugriva as the king and Angad as the crown prince.

Rama then told Sugriva, 'Lakshmana will get your coronation ceremony done and I will not enter the city. I shall reside here in Prastravana Hill. It has begun to rain and it will become difficult to travel. We shall resume our search for Sita once the rain stops. You rule your state along with Angad, but remain focused on fulfilling my task as well.' As instructed, Sugriva returned home and Rama stayed back at Prastravana Hill.

The hills were a classic example of scenic beauty. There was a huge quartz rock which served as the seating place for both the brothers. It was raining heavily and they were surrounded with greenery and freshness. The earth was covered with grass and the throaty croaks of frogs could be heard in the distance. The glow-worms lit up the evening sky. The rumble of the clouds further ignited the pangs of longing. Rama was all the more in sorrow, as the weather was goading him to be with his beloved. The ponds and lakes were full to the brim. Fresh leaves had sprouted.

Rama said to Lakshmana, 'The mud in the ponds has settled down and clear water can be seen in the pond. This indicates that the rains are almost over. But still, there is no news of Sita. I just need to find one clue about her whereabouts, and then, if need be, I shall challenge death itself to rescue her.'

He added, 'Sugriva is too occupied with his new-found wealth, power and women. It seems that he has forgotten his promise and lost his focus on the assignment. Do I have to use the same arrow to kill Sugriva which I used to kill Vali? But then, as a monkey does not have moral values, he is wallowing in his wealth and women.'

By now, Lakshmana was welling up with anger and he got up with his bow and arrow to threaten Sugriva.

Rama said, 'Do not kill Sugriva, just scare him enough and bring him to me.'

By then, Hanuman too had realised that Sugriva had forgotten the task of finding the whereabouts of Sita. He took up the issue with Sugriva and using the four tactics of fear, pressure, bribe and punishment (*Saam*, *Daam*, *Dand* and *Bhed*), confronted him. He tried to reason with Sugriva and reminded him of his promise to Lord Rama. Sugriva realised his mistake and told Hanuman that he had fallen prey to the materialistic world, and he should make it up to Rama. He instructed Hanuman to tell all messengers to go and fetch the band of monkeys, wherever they were residing. 'Anyone who is not present within fifteen days shall have to bear my wrath,' he said. At the same time, Lakshmana reached the gates of the city armed with his bow and arrow. He threatened to set the city on fire and destroy everyone. All monkeys got scared and Sugriva too was taken in by the threat. Sugriva told Hanuman to take Tara along and calm Lakshmana down.

Hanuman and Tara approached Lakshmana and after

bowing to him, took him inside the palace. They washed his feet and gave him a comfortable seat.

Sugriva then entered and explained to Lakshmana: 'There is nothing more intoxicating than physical and moral vices; even powerful sages and saints have fallen prey to them. I am just a monkey with far less intellect and knowledge.'

Sugriva, along with Angad and Hanuman, went to Lord Rama and asked for forgiveness.

He said, 'My Lord, how could I, a lowly monkey, be saved of the attraction of your chimerical world, which even the staunchest of saints have fallen prey to?'

Rama said, 'Sugriva, you are as dear to me as Bharata. Now, please take all the steps that will help us find Sita.'

During their conversation, hundreds of monkeys came pouring into the capital, but Rama met each of them.

Sugriva addressed them: 'This is Lord Rama's work. Go and find Sita and return with your findings after one month. Anyone who returns with no news shall be dealt with personally.'

All the monkeys left in search of Sita. A group of monkeys, under the command of Sushen, was sent to the western parts of the land. The northern area was under the command of Shatibal and another group was sent to the East. A team comprising of Neel, Hanuman, Jamvant and Angad, with many other monkeys, was sent in the southern direction.

Sugriva called Hanuman and Angad and advised them to look south. He said, 'Since we had seen the Pushpak Viman carrying Sita fly south, it is quite possible to find her in that region. Go to the southern regions and look for Sita there.'

All bowed down to Sugriva and started their journey as advised. As they were getting ready to leave, Rama called Hanuman and blessed him. He also gave him his ring as a token of love, to hand it over to Sita if he found her.

Rama said to Hanuman, 'You are a good diplomat. Keep working accordingly. When you meet Sita, tell her about our strengths, and to have faith in our rescue mission. We shall come to her soon.'

Hanuman was pleased to be personally instructed and entrusted with the ring by Rama.

The band of monkeys began their search with chants and slogans in praise of Rama. Gradually, each band, from various directions, returned with no news of Sita.

The group of monkeys which had gone southwards, looked for Sita in the forests of the Vindhya Parwat, and then moved further south towards Lodhwan and Saptvarn Chhitwan forest. Jamvant, Hanuman, Angad and their army desperately moved further south, without much success; they began to feel quite hopeless.

The monkeys were looking for Sita everywhere—in the forests, rivers, hills and caves—enquiring from any hermitage they crossed, and slaying any demon that obstructed their path. Hanuman realized that the monkeys were very tired and would soon die of fatigue and thirst if they continued.

Hanuman climbed atop a hill and looked around for water. At a distance, he spotted cranes and swans entering a cave. In the cave, they saw a woman and a hermit. He was meditating. When they reached the cave, the monkeys bowed to the woman.

The female Sage invited them and offered fruits and water. She told them to freshen up. Finally, the lady led them to a narrow tunnel (*bil*). She asked them to shut their eyes and cross the tunnel. She assured them that they would get Sita's whereabouts once they reached the other side of the tunnel. The monkeys did as they were told. They found themselves standing on the sea shore. She told them that this was Vindhyagiri. It had the Prasravan Hill on one side and the great ocean on the other. 'You shall learn the whereabouts of Sita here,' she said.

A lot of time had passed since the monkeys had begun roaming around in search of Sita. They huddled in a group on the side of the Vindhyachal range, and thought of their next move. They also feared that a month had passed and they still had no clue of where Sita could be. Now Sugriva would kill them all, so it would be better if they all killed themselves to escape such a punishment and disgrace.

Angad also thought that since he had been made the crown prince instead of Sugriva, the latter bore some sort of enmity in his heart and would find an excuse to put Angad to death. So it would be better to embrace death here itself. They all unanimously agreed that it was the right thing to do. Then Tar, the great monkey, suggested that they should hide in the Swyamprabha cave; no one would be able to find them there. On the other hand, Hanuman thought that since most of the monkeys were in favour of Angad, it was quite possible that they would sow seeds of dissent and form their own rival group against Sugriva,

*The Slaying of Vali* ❦ 65

have him assassinated and place Angad on the throne.

Hanuman was dedicated to Sugriva as Sugriva was the God-son of Surya. Surya had accepted Hanuman as his pupil. After completing his education, Hanuman had asked Surya what he desired as *guru dakshina* (or a teacher's fees). The Sun-god had turned down the request.

On Hanuman's insistence, he had said, 'Sugriva is my son and I want you to look after him, always.'

It was because of this promise that Hanuman went to Sugriva and lived with him. When Sugriva ran to Rishimukh Hill, he ran with him.

Hanuman had applied all means (Saam, Daam, Dand and Bhed) to force Angad to align with Sugriva in the search for Sita. Angad was intelligent, powerful and was adorned with all virtues.

Four principles are required to achieve someone's support for the completion of a task. Hanuman, who knew all the laws and arts of politics and had outstanding oratory skills, polarized the monkeys and Angad, and convinced them to stay together.

The army of monkeys decided that they would not return till they found out about Sita. They all sipped the ocean's water (*aachaman*) and vowed to find Sita or end their lives there on the seaside.

Jamvant tried to encourage the group. He said, 'Do not take Rama to be an ordinary person. He is the Lord incarnate. We are fortunate to be offered the opportunity to serve him'.

In one of the caves in the hill stayed the Vulture King Sampati. Hearing the howls and shrieks of the monkeys, he felt happy and thought aloud, 'The Lord has provided me with food at my doorstep. How lucky I am! I shall have a meal to my heart's content.'

He came out of his cave. As soon as the monkeys saw him, they all got scared. Jamvant wondered what should be done. Angad planned to divert Sampati's attention and said loudly, 'No one can be as great as Jatayu. He gave up his life just to help Lord Rama and found a place in heaven.'

Hearing Jatayu's name, Sampati reassured Angad that he meant no harm to them. He further asked Angad to tell him more about Jatayu. Angad told him the entire story and praised the Lord. After hearing the story, Sampati said: 'I know about Sita. My son had told me about her.'

Sampati further said, 'My brother Jatayu gave up his life trying to save Sita. I am old but featherless. Please take me to the seashore. After offering my last tribute to my departed brother, I shall give you the details about Sita.'

The monkeys helped the old Sampati to the seashore. He offered Jatayu the *Tilanjali*, or an oblation of a handful of water, with sesame seeds, to the deceased. After that the monkeys brought him back to his resting place. They requested him to reveal everything he knew about Sita. Sampati said, 'I have very sharp eyesight. I can see Ravana and Sita across the sea.'

Sampati continued, 'Now I shall tell you how I learnt about Sita's whereabouts.' He said: 'I burnt my wings flying too close to the Sun out of pride. Since then, I spend most of my time lying here. My son, Suparshav, took care of me and brought my daily meals. Vultures are known to have an insatiable hunger.

'One day, I was very hungry. I wanted to eat something desperately. My son had gone out to hunt, but he returned after sunset and that too, empty-handed. I was very angry at him. He told me politely that while he was standing on the peak of the Mahendra Hills, he saw a man, with dark complexion, carrying a woman. My son decided to grab them for our meals. But then, the man very humbly requested my son to let them pass. He spoke so humbly and gently that my son decided to let them go. That is why he got delayed and did not bring anything to eat.

'That man was Ravana and the lady was Sita, whom he had thought of grabbing as our meals. They have gone to Lanka. The Trikut Hill is across the ocean and Lanka at its peak. Ravana, the King of Lanka, is a strong warrior. In his garden, Sita is sitting at Ashok Vatika. I can see her from here, but you cannot. You should now go ahead and fulfil the task assigned to you by your Lord.

'I could have helped you had I not been so old. Only someone who can leap across this ocean of a hundred leagues, or *yojan*, will be able to fulfil Rama's mission.'

Sampati then looked at himself and exclaimed, 'Look! As told by Rishi Chandrama, how my new feathers have started to grow. You too should take the Lord's name and start your search. You shall definitely find Sita.' Sampati then took their leave, leaving the monkeys to plan their next move.

The monkeys gathered around Angad and discussed their respective ability to jump across the ocean. They also suggested that Angad should come up with a plan to cross the ocean of a hundred leagues. However, they failed to reach a conclusion.

Jamvant said, 'Now I am very old and fatigued and have no strength at all. Otherwise, I could have jumped across the ocean without a second thought.'

Angad said, 'I will be able to reach the other shore, but I am not sure if I will be able to come back.'

Jamvant said: 'Angad, you are powerful and full of virtues, but you are also our leader. How can you leave under such circumstances?'

Jamvant then turned to Hanuman and said, 'Hanuman, you are the son of the wind God. Why are you silent? What are you thinking? You are virtually a mine of intelligence, wits and science. Your strength equals the power of the wind. You can achieve everything in this world.'

Jamvant encouraged Hanuman and said, 'As a child you were very powerful, intelligent and inquisitive. You used to ask a lot of questions and trouble the rishis on not getting appropriate answers. When it became unbearable, they cursed you to forget your own strengths and power, only to remember them when someone reminds you of your potential. Once again, you will become invincible.'

He continued: 'Let me tell you the story of your birth... Sage Kashyap was pleased with Kesri, your father, and asked him what he desired. Kesri said, "If you are really happy with me, give me a son as powerful and mighty as God Marut (wind)."

'The sage said, "So be it."

'That is how you were born to Anjana Devi. At the time of your birth, Pawan Dev, the Wind God, came and said that you shall be as mighty as him.

'Once, you grabbed the Sun and put it in your mouth. There was darkness all around and all the Gods pleaded with you to release the Sun. Lord Indra was very angry with your action, and he struck you with a thunderbolt. You fell unconscious with the strike and your chin was broken. Pawan Dev got very angry, and stopped the wind from flowing.

'The gods told Pawan Dev to ask for whatever he desired, but not stop the air from flowing. Pawan Dev asked for undisputed strength, might, courage and a clever mind for you, Hanuman. He also demanded that you remain a devotee of Lord Rama. Ganesha said that just like him, you too shall have the powers to remove all hurdles in your path.

'Lord Shiva blessed you, saying that you shall be a *Mritunjaya*, or one who is victorious over death, like himself. Lord Brahma blessed you with *Bajrangi*—a body which is stronger than the thunderbolt (mace) of Lord Indra. You will also not be affected by the supreme weapon of Brahma, the "Brahmastra". Lord Brahma, on behalf of all the gods, blessed you and said that devotion to you is enough to please all the gods. Since your chin is deformed due to Indra's blow, you were to be called Hanuman.'

Hanuman remembered all his virtues after listening to the story and said, 'Please be patient, do not be sad. I am the servant of Lord Rama. I accept the responsibility of going to Lanka and bringing back news of Sita.' All the monkeys cheered for Hanuman. Angad was relieved that they would be able to complete the work they were assigned.

Hanuman roared and grew in size to be as huge as a mountain. He said, 'I shall jump across the ocean. This is child's play. I shall vanquish Ravana, along with his entire army, and bring the whole Trikut Hill here across the ocean.'

He then requested Jamvant to guide him through this mission. Jamvant said: 'Do not get overexcited. Just go, and bring us news about Sita; we shall inform Lord Rama. It is up to him to form an army and win over Lanka and bring Sita back safely. He is self-sufficient for this job. He has the capability to kill Ravana alone, but he will take the army of apes to pressurize him.'

Hanuman was pleased by Jamvant's words. He addressed his fellow soldiers: 'Brothers, you will wait here. I shall soon return with news about Mother Sita. I am sure this mission shall be successful.' So saying, Hanuman bade farewell to his friends and left for Lanka.

There was a hillock on the seashore. Hanuman climbed it effortlessly. On reaching the top, Hanuman jumped on the peak and it sunk to the netherworld. The ocean reminded the hill Mainak: 'Since Pawan Dev had helped you once, you need to return the favour. You should be a resting place for Hanuman (Pawan Putra).' On this advice, Mainak rose from the ocean bed and requested Hanuman to take rest for a while on its crust.

Hanuman, offering salutations, said, 'Thank you for being so considerate, but I cannot rest until I have accomplished the task assigned to me by my Lord,' and moved forward.

To test Hanuman's strength and intelligence, the gods

sent in Soorsa, the mother of the serpents. She appeared in front of Hanuman and said: 'The Gods have sent me a tasty dish today.'

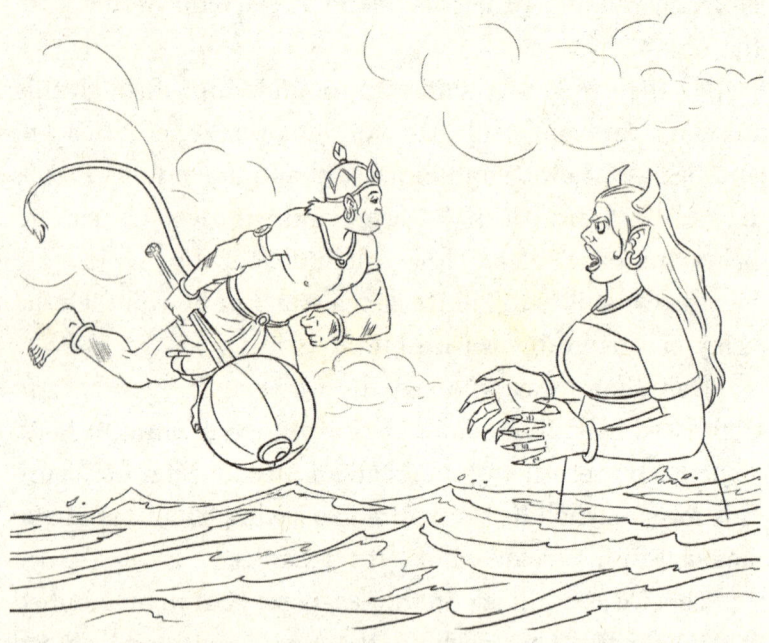

Hanuman pleaded with folded hands: 'Mother, please let me go today, I am on my Lord's mission. Let me convey to him the news about Mother Sita, and then I shall myself return and sit in your mouth and you can have me as your meal.' But Soorsa was adamant.

Finally, Hanuman said, 'If you are not willing to listen, then why don't you eat me?'

Hearing this, Soorsa opened her mouth wide. Hanuman grew bigger and bigger. She opened her mouth to a league's width, but Hanuman grew double that size. When Soorsa increased her mouth to sixteen leagues, Hanuman grew twice as much. No matter how wide Soorsa opened her mouth, Hanuman kept doubling his size to that. Finally, when she opened her mouth wide enough to accommodate 100 leagues, Hanuman turned himself into a very tiny monkey and entered and came out of Soorsa's mouth before she could close it. He then bowed and took her leave. Soorsa said that the gods had sent her to test his wit and intelligence, and he had proven himself. She also blessed him for the successful completion of the task. Hanuman continued on his journey.

There lived a demoness, Simhika, in the ocean. With her power to cast illusions, she could suck and swallow the birds flying in the sky just with the help of their shadow. She tried the same deception with Hanuman when he was flying across the ocean, but Hanuman saw through her deceit. He killed her and reached the other side of the ocean.

He saw beautiful gardens with fruit laden trees and flowers of various hues and smell on the other side. Bees were hovering over the flowers and the entire ambiance was of sublime beauty and tranquillity. Moving further, he came across a high hill top. He climbed over it and saw Lanka. There he saw a very beautiful golden palace. It was a breathtaking view, with spires and domes painted with gold. It was surrounded by the ocean on all sides. It had numerous gardens and orchards all around and was also dotted with quite a few arenas. The city was guarded from all sides. Hanuman thought that he would transform himself into a tiny being and enter the city after nightfall.

At nightfall, Hanuman reduced himself to the size of

a mosquito and entered Lanka. The gates of Lanka were guarded by a demoness, Lankini.

She saw Hanuman and asked him, 'Where are you going without paying me regards? I am the gatekeeper of Lanka and do not allow anyone to enter without my permission. I eat anyone who tries to enter the gates without permission.'

Hanuman struck her with a mighty blow. She started bleeding through her mouth and fell down on the ground. She staggered to her feet and with folded hands, told Hanuman, 'After blessing Ravana, Lord Brahma told me that when you fall after a strike by a monkey, you should understand that your rakshas days are nearing an end. The demons will be vanquished. Now, I am fortunate that I had the privilege to see the messenger of Lord Rama. Go, in the name of the Lord, and complete your task.'

Reducing himself to his miniscule form, Hanuman entered the city. He peeped into every house to look for Sita. He also entered Ravana's palace to look for her, but he did not find Sita anywhere.

During the search, he came near the beautiful palace. In the palace, there was a temple with the symbol of Rama's bow inscribed on it. Outside the temple was a tulsi (basil) plant. He got enthusiastic on seeing the temple. He wondered who this saintly man in this city of demons could be. Just then, he heard the slogan, 'Rama, Rama'. Hanuman was even more pleased. He had found a devotee of Rama in this foreign land inhabited by demons. He thought that a saintly person should always be helpful rather than being a trouble-maker. So he immediately made up his mind to befriend this saintly person. Hanuman, in the guise of a Brahmin, went to Vibhishana's door and chanted 'Rama-Rama'. Vibhishana immediately came out and bowed down to the Brahmin and asked the purpose of his visit. He said, 'You seem to be a devotee of the Lord and I ingratiate myself by your presence.' Hanuman narrated the entire story to him. Vibhishana said, 'I am staying in this land just like the tongue stays in between the teeth. I am a person who is prone to "tamo gun" (virtues of tamas/anger/tamsik); I also have no control over my senses or feelings. Will Lord Rama bestow his favours and benevolence on a person like me? I feel that without the blessings of a saint one cannot get close to the Lord.'

Hanuman replied, 'The Lord is always affectionate towards his devotees. I am a monkey of a temperamental nature. If someone sees my face in the morning, he will be repulsed and might not be able to eat the entire day, but with Shri Rama's blessings it is not so now.'

Vibhishana then intimated Hanuman about Sita and how she was passing each day painfully, yearning for her Lord Rama. Hanuman expressed his desire to meet Sita. Vibhishana told him of a plan and how to execute it.

# The Lankan Inferno

Hanuman then took his leave of Vibhishana and entered Ashok Vatika, where Sita had been staying, as a tiny monkey. Ashok Vatika is also known as Pamadavan. Hanuman watched Sita, hiding behind a tree. She seemed miserable and stared at her feet, muttering the name of Lord Rama in her heart. Seeing her in such a desolate state, Hanuman felt very sad. He sat there amidst branches and leaves and thought of his next step. Just then, Ravana entered the Ashok Vatika and approached Sita. Ravana was accompanied with several women dressed up in the finest clothes. Mandodari, Ravana's wife, was also there with him.

Ravana tried all sorts of tactics to reason with Sita to accept his advances. He said, 'Oh my doe-eyed, dear one! I shall make Mandodari and my other queens your servants. Just look at me with love in your eyes.' Sita tried to avoid his gaze by placing a small twig in their line of sight and uttered the name of Lord Rama.

Then, she replied, 'Ravana, you are not aware of the powers of Shri Rama's arrows. Just as the Kumudani (lily) flower does not blossom in the light of the glow worm, you shall never be able to change my mind. You did not have the courage to confront Rama. You used deception to abduct me. Are you not ashamed of your deeds?'

Ravana became furious when he heard Sita compare

him to a glow worm and Rama to the Sun. He screamed at her, 'Sita, you have insulted me. I shall cut your head off with my Chandrahasa sword if you do not accept my terms.'

Sita replied, 'Only Rama's arms will adorn my neck as a garland. Either that, or I accept this sword. In fact, I pray to this sword to free me of the suffering caused by the separation from my Lord. Its sharp edge shall be my relief.'

Ravana rushed towards Sita with the sword in his hand, but Mandodari stopped him and said that killing her will not be the right thing to do. Ravana called for the demonesses who were guarding Sita and ordered them to make Sita accept his wishes in one month's time, or he would chop off her head. He marched off to his palace and the demonesses started tormenting Sita.

One of the demonesses guarding Sita was Trijita. She was very clever and a devotee of Lord Rama. She called the other demonesses on duty and said, 'I had a dream where a monkey sets Lanka on fire. All the demons were killed and Ravana was made to sit on a donkey without clothes. His ten heads shaved and twenty arms chopped off. He was moving south and Vibhishana was to become the King of Lanka. The entire city was reverberating with cries of 'long live Lord Rama, victory to Shri Rama, salute to Shri Rama' and singing his praises. Finally, I saw Rama taking Sita back to the palace. I am telling the truth. This dream shall come true within a few days. Be good to Sita by serving her so that you are in her good books. When the time comes, you shall be spared from any punishment.' The demonesses were scared and they all fell on Sita's feet and asked for forgiveness. Then they scattered in all directions.

Sita was scared that Ravana would kill her in a month's time. She begged Trijita to help her pass this tough time. She asked her to suggest a way she could end her miserable life. She was tired of waiting and the torture inflicted upon her. She asked Trijita to bring some wood and prepare a pyre, which she would enter. Trijita would then set it alight.

Trijita, to divert Sita's mind, said, 'It is very late now. How can I arrange for any wood and fire at this time? Think of your Lord and his valiant deeds.' The demoness then went back to her home.

Hanuman got worried on seeing Sita lament. Hidden, he dropped the ring that Rama had given to him in front of her. Sita picked it up and recognized the ring as it read 'Rama'. Joy and sorrow engulfed her as she thought Rama was close by. She wondered where the ring came from. It could not be an illusion. Did that mean that someone had defeated him and taken it? But then, if he was invincible, how could he be defeated?

At that moment, Hanuman started praising of the Lord. He, still in hiding, narrated the whole story of what had happened till now. Sita called out aloud: 'Whoever is narrating this story, why don't you appear before me?'

Hanuman came down from his hiding place and stood before Sita. She turned her face away at the sight of Hanuman.

Hanuman said, 'Mother, please do not look away. I swear upon the Lord, I am his messenger. I am the one who has brought this ring. Lord Rama has sent this for you to assure you that you will be rescued soon.' Sita was bewildered and asked, 'How can a human and a monkey be friends?'

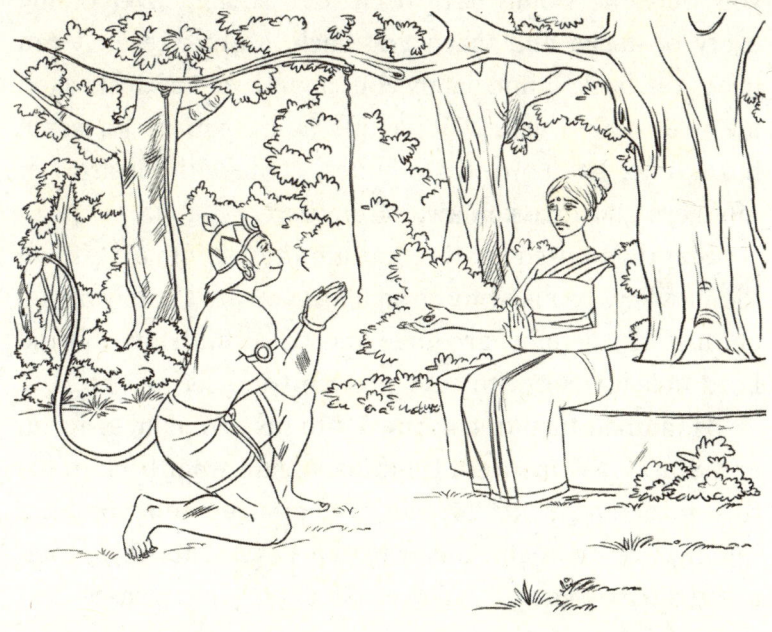

Hanuman then told her how Sugriva was made king. He also told her that Sugriva, under the guidance of Lord Rama, had sent monkeys in all directions in search of her. 'I, along with other monkeys, came to the south, and now I have come to Ashok Vatika.'

She then asked Hanuman, 'How are my Lord and his brother? Why have they left me at the mercy of these demons? Will I ever be able to meet them again?'

Hanuman tried to reassure her and said, 'Lord Rama and his brother are very as well. Rama loves you immensely. Rama once said, "Your grief reduces if you share it with someone. But I have no one to share my grief with. As such, only I have to bear it".'

Hanuman further said, 'Had the Lord known where you were, he would have been here sooner, overcoming every obstacle, and taken you back. Mother, even I can take you back immediately, but my Lord has instructed me to just find you. Mother, please be patient for some more time. The Lord will definitely come with his army of monkeys and take you away from here.'

Sita then posed another question to Hanuman: 'Are all the monkeys in his army as small as you are? I am worried because the demons are huge and powerful. How will the Lord defeat them with such an army and set me free?'

Hanuman then transformed into his divine, huge form, and Sita was convinced. Hanuman again went back to his tiny form and said, 'Mother, we monkeys do not have intelligence or might, but with the Lord's blessings, even a snake can defeat a vulture.' Sita was very pleased and blessed Hanuman.

She said that he was the epitome of might and intelligence. He would be immortal. Hanuman was very happy to get Sita's blessings.

Hanuman then said to Sita, 'Mother, I am hungry. With your permission, I would like to eat some fruits.'

Sita said, 'Son, this garden is heavily guarded by mighty demons; they could hurt you.'

Hanuman said, 'Mother, if you permit me, I will not fear the demons.'

Sita said, 'Then it is OK, son. Go ahead!'

Hanuman bowed to Sita and took her leave. He entered

the orchards surrounding the garden. He ate a few fruits and then started uprooting the trees. He also killed a few demons who tried to stop him. Some of them managed to save themselves and ran to Ravana crying for help.

They told Ravana, 'Lord, a huge monkey has entered the gardens. He has been eating the fruits and uprooting the trees. He has devastated the entire Ashok Vatika. He has crushed many of our comrades under his feet and killed them.'

Ravana sent some more soldiers, whom Hanuman killed instantly. Those who could save themselves, ran to Ravana again. He then sent his youngest son Akshaykumar with five commanders—Virupaksh, Upaksh, Durdhar, Pradhan, and Bhaskarn. Prahastra's son Jaambumali, and seven sons of his brave ministers, were also sent. Hanuman killed all the demons. He also killed Akshaykumar. Hearing this, Ravana asked his son, Meghnad, to go and get Hanuman. He said, 'Son, do not kill the monkey, but get him here alive.'

Meghnad rushed out in rage towards Ashok Vatika. Hanuman uprooted a huge tree and smashed it on Meghnad's chariot which broke to pieces. After killing all the demons who had accompanied Meghnad, Hanuman turned his attention towards Meghnad. He struck Meghnad with a mighty blow and climbed up a tree. Meghnad fell unconscious. He was unable to tackle Hanuman with his might and deceit. He then attacked Hanuman with the Brahmastra, the weapon of Lord Brahma. The Brahmastra had no effect on him as Brahma himself had blessed Hanuman with immunity against it. However, Hanuman thought that if he neutralised the weapon, its very essence would be belittled and its reputation would be vanquished.

In deference to Lord Brahma, Hanuman fell unconscious as soon as he was struck by the weapon. Meghnad tied him up with the Naagpash and carried him to Ravana's assembly hall. The demons rushed to catch a glimpse of the monkey who had been tormenting them.

Ravana was furious due to the loss of his son. He spoke harshly with Hanuman and ridiculed him.

He asked Hanuman, 'Who are you? Why did you kill the demons? Do you not fear for your life?'

Hanuman replied, 'I am Hanuman, the messenger of Lord Rama. I know you too. You had once fought with Sahastrabahu. But what could I have done? I was hungry. Being a monkey, it is my nature to climb trees, eat their fruits and break them. I beat up and killed only those who tried to attack me. And that is why your son, Meghnad, has brought me here, tied up like this. I have no problems in being tied up but I want to carry on with my Lord's errand. So please, listen to me. Return Sita to my Lord. Rama is very noble. He will forgive you, if you accept his protection. You can then rule over Lanka without any problem. Please do not stain the noble clan of Sage Pulastya.'

Hearing Hanuman's words, Ravana mocked him. 'It seems that now I have found a very intelligent teacher!'

He then warned Hanuman that his end was near. Hanuman retorted, 'It is the other way around. My end isn't near, but yours is. Rama and Sugriva are neither gods nor Gandharvas, they are neither Yakshas nor Asuras. Rama is a human and Sugriva is an ape. And as per Brahma's boon, you can only be killed by a human or by an animal. How will you save yourself from them? Killing Vali, slaying demons, and his friendship with Sugriva—all point in one direction for Rama. You should think it over and draw your own conclusions.'

Ravana got very angry and told Hanuman that he had lost his mind. He then asked the court, 'Why does not someone get rid of this monkey?'

Ravana announced that Hanuman was to be executed. The news spread like wildfire all over the city. Vibhishana rushed to the assembly hall with a few of his ministers.

Vibhishana told Ravana that it is against the law to execute a messenger. Ravana retorted, 'I know it is against ethics to kill a messenger, but then, messengers do not wage war on their visits. He has waged a war against my soldiers. So, he shall be punished.'

Vibhishana insisted that Hanuman must not have started the fight. He only retaliated in self-defence. He requested Ravana to not execute him. If he must, punish him in some other way. 'If you want to show your strength to your enemy, send your army with few powerful warriors to capture the princes,' he said.

Ravana then said, 'Dismember him. Monkeys love their tails. Wrap a cloth around his tail and set it on fire.'

Hanuman was not perturbed. He thought to himself that when he came to the city the previous night, he could not see the city properly. Now when they would set his tail on fire, he would light up the whole city and be able to see its layout and the fort properly. This would help them plan their next move and also the attack.

On Ravana's instruction, *ghee* (clarified butter), oil and cloth were arranged. Hanuman's tail grew longer and longer. The entire city's oil and ghee were exhausted. To celebrate, the residents came out beating drums and cymbals. They took Hanuman around the city. Then, they put his tail on fire. Hanuman suddenly transformed himself into a smaller form. He jumped from one building to another. To assist his son, the wind also blew hard, spreading the fire across the city. Soon, the entity of Lanka was burning. Only Vibhishana's house remained safe from this fire.

However, instead of getting charred, the city began to shine. When gold is subjected to heat, its sheen increases and it becomes purer. Hanuman was confused. He pondered why was Lanka not getting charred. Just then, he spotted someone hanging upside down from a tree with his back towards Lanka. He asked him, 'Who are you?'

He replied, 'I am Shani Dev (Lord Saturn). Ravana has imprisoned me and has hung me from this tree. Please free me and once I set my gaze on Lanka, it will be charred. (It is believed that when Lord Saturn sets his gaze on anything, it burns, unable to withstand the power of the gaze.) Hanuman set Saturn free. He looked upon Lanka. The gleam vanished and Lanka stood black and charred.

Lord Saturn was indebted to Hanuman for setting him free and so it is believed that whosoever has the blessings of Hanuman, is never troubled by Lord Saturn.

After setting Lanka on fire, Hanuman jumped into the ocean and doused his tail. He thought to himself, 'By burning Lanka, I have committed what is called "monkey-mischief". I have done something which is not right. I have done Adharm (sin). If Mother Sita has been hurt in this fire, I would have committed double the mistakes by not adhering to the task I was reposed with.' He tried to reassure himself by thinking that maybe Mother Sita was safe from the fire by her own divinity.'

Meanwhile, Hanuman heard the words of praises from the bards and sages. They said that he had accomplished a wonderful task. He was happy and understood that Mother Sita was safe, or peoples' reactions would have been different.

Hanuman then rested for a while. He took his tiny form and went back to Sita. But he was feeling uneasy because of the heat. Sita applied a vermillion paste, or *sindoor*, on his body, which had a very soothing effect. Since then, Hanuman's body has always been depicted in red.

Hanuman said to Sita, 'Mother, Lord Rama had given me a ring to be handed over to you as a proof that it was him who sent me to you. Similarly, you too must give me a token of your identity for Rama.'

Sita took off a piece of jewellery from her hair called *Choodamani* and gave it to Hanuman. She told him to offer the Lord her salutations. She said, 'Lord, please set me free from this dangerous and scary place.'

She further said to Hanuman, 'Earlier, I had been feeling the pangs of separation, but now after meeting you, I am at peace. Now that you have to leave, my fears are returning. Please go and tell my Lord that if he does not come within a month's time, I will kill myself.'

Hanuman reassured Sita, 'Please be patient. Rama will definitely come.'

He then prepared for his journey back to Lord Rama. On his way back, he came across Mainak, the hillock. But in his eagerness to convey the good news to his Lord as early as possible, he again refused to rest. He just touched Mainak and offered his salutations. On reaching the Mahandragiri Hills on the northern coast, he let out a deafening roar. His friends on the other side heard his roar and were assured of his safe arrival and good news.

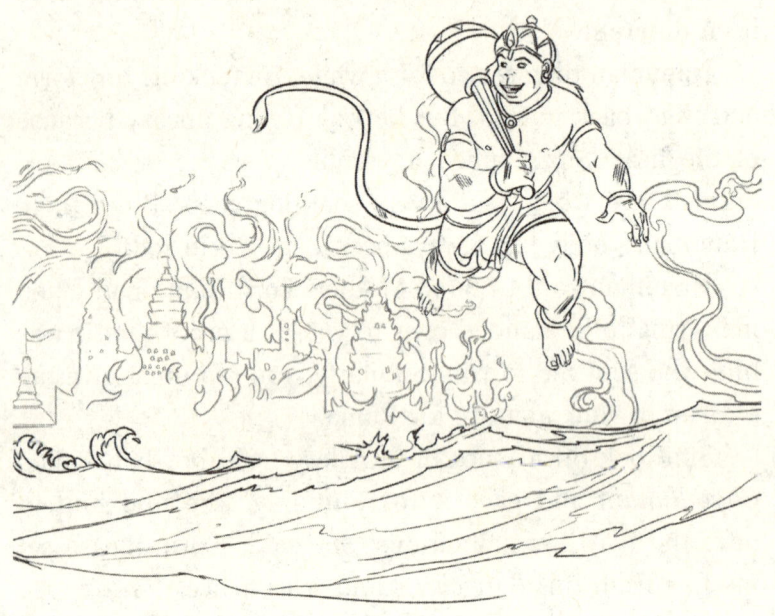

When Hanuman reached the other side, everyone was happy to see him and the smile on his face indicated that he had been successful in completing the Lord's mission.

Hanuman then narrated the incidents which took place in Lanka. Angad said that they should now attack Lanka and defeat the demons, set Sita free and take her to Lord Rama. But Jamvant objected to this plan. He said that taking any action without Rama's consent would be wrong. Everyone agreed with Jamvant and they started their journey back to Kishkindha. They chatted jubilantly all the way about new ideas and plans of action. With Angad's permission, they stopped at Madhuban to taste fresh fruits. Madhuban was Sugriva's beautiful and idyllic garden, equal to Indra's Nandan Van. It was under the protection of Sugriva's maternal uncle, Mahavir Dadhimukh. Dadhimukh objected to this, but he was harassed by the monkeys. The two groups—Dadhimukh's and Hanuman's—engaged in a pitched battle. Dadhimukh complained to Sugriva about the monkeys' behaviour. Sugriva, sensing the mood, was also amused and guessed that they must have brought good news. However, the monkeys had damaged the garden in their excitement. A little later, the group reached Sugriva and informed him that Hanuman had successfully completed the mission. Sugriva came and met Hanuman and then took everyone to Lord Rama.

Rama and Lakshmana were sitting on the quartz rock when the monkeys came and fell at Rama's feet. Rama enquired about the wellbeing of each one. Jamvant then said, 'Lord, Hanuman has completed your task successfully. How he did it is beyond words!'

Hearing this, Lord Rama embraced Hanuman and asked him, 'Brother, Where is Janaki? How is she taking care of herself amongst the demons there?'

Hanuman said, 'Mother has given me this choodamani as a token for you.' Rama took the choodamani and held it to his chest.

Hanuman conveyed Sita's message to Rama: 'You, being the remover of all worries and disorders of the universe, how have you forgotten me? My affection and love for you is three-fold. I love you with *manas, vacha* and *karmana* (body, mind and soul). Yes, I do agree that I am at fault at one level. In your absence, even now, how am I alive? I can only say that my eyes were so eager to see you that my soul could not leave the body. My body was as delicate as a ball of cotton and the pangs of separation acted like fire, to destroy me. But it was my eyes, which were patiently waiting for you. They kept on a steady stream of tears that doused the fire.'

Hanuman then requested Rama, 'Lord, please hurry and fetch Mother Sita. She is in a lot of pain.'

Rama's eyes welled up with tears. He said to Hanuman, 'Hanuman, you have completed the task with perfection. I shall always be indebted to you. Tell me, what can I do for you?'

Hanuman fell at Rama's feet. Rama helped him to get up and asked, 'How did you set Lanka on fire?'

Hanuman humbly replied, 'Lord, how can I, a monkey, accomplish such a great feat. I, being a monkey, kept leaping from one place to another. The rest was the miracle of your divine powers.'

Rama then called for Sugriva and said, 'Prepare your army. Gather everybody and summon all the monkeys and bears. There should be no delay.'

Hanuman apprised Rama of the layout of the city of Lanka. He described in detail the main gate, army barracks, security arrangements and the fort. He also described the special draw bridge and the moat surrounding the fort. He told Rama that when the enemy is on the bridge, it turns over and the enemies fall into the gorge. Hanuman further explained that there are four main gates to Lanka and each gate is heavily guarded by demons with weapons like cannons and four-feet long maces with iron spikes. Hanuman also told Rama that he had already destroyed the draw bridge and vanquished a quarter of Ravana's army.

Hanuman narrated Ravana's strategy and the organizing capacity which he had applied to expand his kingdom. Ravana had brought together the demons, rakshasas, mutants and asurs under one umbrella, to have unity amongst the non-human class, and combine their powers. His organizing strategy was a culture in itself, and is known as 'Rakshsanskriti' or Demon culture.

The basic foundation of this culture was 'Vayam Rakshami'—those under this tutelage are given full protection by Ravana. 'Vayam Rakshami' literally means 'I will protect'. In a broader sense, it means protection and provision of all and anything that is required. Ravana, with his scientific capabilities; had invented rare weapons of war, and his soldiers were armed with them. Thus, he had an upper hand on the battlefield. He was always present on the battlefield. He strategized and supervised the attacks. So, before taking on Ravana, it is imperative that one should first understand his ten basic virtues.

All commanders, along with Sugriva, came and bowed before Lord Rama. Rama, along with everyone, prepared to go to the seashore. Rama said, 'The afternoon is an auspicious time for victory—Vijay Mahurat—but at this time any journey towards the south is prohibited. Lanka is to the south-east of Kishkindha. We shall proceed to the afternoon.'

At the appointed time, the army moved forward. Many auspicious signs filled the atmosphere. In Lanka, Sita also witnessed similar auspicious signs. In contrast, Ravana experienced the exact opposite.

The weapons of Rama's army, which comprises of monkeys and bears, were nails and claws. With loud growls and roars, they chanted Lord Rama's name and hailed victory. They moved forward and reached the seashore. They spread out in different directions and started feeding on fruits and other edibles available in the area.

Since the time Hanuman had set Lanka afire, the women of Lanka were scared. They all wondered that if the messenger was so powerful, what the Lord would be like. And when his entire army comes to invade Lanka, what would be the outcome? The inputs from her informers also aroused fear and apprehension in Mandodari. She visited her husband and advised him against starting a war.

She told him to return Sita to Rama and forge a truce. Mandodari told Ravana that even if Brahma and Shiva wanted to help him, they would be helpless as long as he did not return Sita to Rama. Ravana mocked Mandodari and said, 'Women are by nature timid. The demons will eat up all the monkeys.'

He then embraced Mandodari and said, 'You are Ravana's wife, and even then you are afraid. This is not right!'

Vibhishana was a Rama devotee and he too was not in favour of keeping Sita as a prisoner in Ashok Vatika and coercing her for marriage. Vibhishana was a man of integrity, principles and intelligence. He also tried to reason with Ravana, but the King did not pay any attention to what Vibhishana said.

When Ravana reached his court the next day, he was informed that the army of monkeys had reached the seashores on the other side of the ocean. Ravana was least bothered, partly because of his arrogance and partly due to his ministers' assurances that the apes did not stand a chance against the one who had vanquished the gods.

It will be the end of religion, body and State if teachers, doctors and ministers, respectively, wrongly advice their people. If their advice is right and they are not followed, the effect on the State and religion will be same. Here, in this case, Ravana did not listen to Vibhishana and Mandodari, but heeded his ministers who were wrong. This clearly indicated that the end of Ravana was not far away.

This madness was greatly responsible for taking Ravana to his end. At that moment, Vibhishana entered the assembly hall and took his seat.

Ravana asked Vibhishana, 'What have you to say?'

Vibhishana stood up and said, 'If you are asking for my opinion, I shall speak only what shall be good for you. If you are interested in your wellbeing, I would suggest returning Sita, with all respect, to her husband Rama. Lust, greed, anger and arrogance—all lead to hell. Leave all this and chant the name of Lord Rama. Return Sita to Rama and he will forgive you.' Sage Pulastya also gave the same advice to Ravana through one of his messengers.

Malyavant, who was on of Ravana's ministers, was well known for his intelligence and unbiased attitude. He said, 'Lord, what your brother Vibhishana is saying is the best course of action, and you should follow his suggestion.'

But arrogant Ravaan asked his soldiers to throw them out of the court. Malyavant quietly got up and left the hall.

Vibhishana once again tried to persuade Ravana. He said, 'Humans possess intelligence and foolishness in equal quantities. Where there is intelligence, there is prosperity, but where there is foolishness, the result of the deed is always unfortunate. The foolishness that is in your heart at the moment with respect to Sita is surely the death knell for the demons. You are blinded by your foolishness and are unable to see beyond it. You are unable to see the end of demons. Brother, I urge you once again to return Sita.' Vibhishana's advice, which was in line with the teachings of all the Vedas and the righteous path of living, offended Ravana.

He shouted at Vibhishana, 'Your end is near. You live with me and bear a liking and respect to sages and saints? You are living on my mercy but are sympathetic towards my enemies.'

Ravana kicked Vibhishana and shouted, 'Go and seek refuge with the enemy.' Vibhishana, still, clung to Ravana's feet and pleaded, 'You are like my father. I would not mind even if you beat me, but I would request you to please settle the issue with Rama and sign a truce.'

Vibhishana then said, 'Your assembly is in the grip of death. I am going into Lord Rama's shelter. Do not blame me for your devastation and the ultimate annihilation of the demon race.'

Vibhishana walked out of Ravana's court along with his four loyal ministers, Anal, Anil, Har, and Sampati. The moment Vibhishana, the embodiment of religion, walked out of Lanka, the empire moved another step closer to its end.

On his way out, he thought of this as a moment of happiness. He was going to see the Lord, the mere touch of whose feet had turned a stone into a woman. It was fortunate to get a chance to touch the same feet. Vibhishana reached the other side of the ocean. The monkeys saw them and wondered what brought them there. They took them to be informants sent to spy on their preparations. They stopped Vibhishana on the seashore and informed Sugriva. Sugriva then told Rama of Vibhishana's arrival.

Rama spoke with everyone and asked for their opinions. Sugriva said that one could never be sure of the demons' intentions. They could not ascertain what the demons had come for. The demons should be taken as prisoners.

Angad said, 'Since they have come from the enemies' camp, we need to be wary. We should arrive at a conclusion only after interrogating them.'

Finally, Hanuman said, 'Lord, you are omniscient. But keeping in mind the present situation, I would say that he must have heard about your illustrious past. He must have heard how you helped Sugriva get his kingdom back after killing his brother Vali. It appears that he has come with a similar proposal—to get his share of the kingdom after defeating Ravana. He must have carefully weighed the consequences of seeking help from you. I feel it would help us if we have him on our side.'

Rama said, 'What you have said is correct, and we must always help those who come to us for support.'

Hearing Rama's words, Sugriva said, 'One who can betray his brother can betray anyone!'

Rama said, 'It is the close relatives, friends and brothers who betray the most in the time of any need. It is this fear that has brought Vibhishana to us. Moreover, neither are all brothers like Bharata, nor are all sons like me; neither are all friends like you, Sugriva.' Sugriva, hearing this, still maintained that it would be safer if they held Vibhishana as a prisoner, but agreed to Rama's suggestion of including Vibhishana into their fold.

On Rama's instructions, Angad and Hanuman, along with some other apes, went to fetch Vibhishana with full honour. They brought them to Rama. Vibhishana bowed to the princes and said, 'I am Vibhishana, Ravana's brother, and have come to you for shelter and protection. Please save me.' Rama gave Vibhishana a seat near him and asked, 'How are you, Lankesh (King of Lanka)?'

Rama said, 'You are clever and a strategist as well. Your feelings are never unjust. You have been living with demons and lawless people. Tell me, how could you nurture your true self? I knew about you and your ethics. I believe that it is easier to live in hell than with a wicked person. I understand that you may not have greed for the throne of Lanka, but even then, just meeting me and asking for my shelter has its benefits. It is impossible that my blessings will not bear fruits. You shall certainly have something beneficial coming your way.' Rama applied tilak on Vibhishana's forehead, proclaiming him the King of Lanka. The bounty that Ravana had earned after sacrificing his ten heads to Lord Shiva was given to Vibhishana without much ado. He deserved much more.

It is believed that Rama had a special affection for Vibhishana. It was because of this affection that, despite everyone's reluctance, Rama welcomed Vibhishana.

To give further importance and leverage to Vibhishana, Rama, the omniscient and the destroyer of demons on Earth, asked him, 'Tell us, how do we cross the ocean?'

Vibhishana said, 'Your arrows have the power to dry up hundreds of such oceans. But since the ocean is your ancestor, you could request it to show you a way and your army could cross over without any difficulty.'

One of Rama's ancestors was named Sagar. Vibhishana's indication was towards this ancestor. Rama agreed and said, 'Okay, if God is with us, we shall definitely be successful.'

Lakshmana did not favour this soft approach of pleading. He said that one should be sure of his might. It is the weak who call for god's help.

'*Dev dev aalsi pukara*'

He said to Rama, 'You have the power to dry up the ocean just by being angry. Then why plead?'

Rama calmed him down and said, 'Be patient,

Lakshmana. I shall do exactly that.'

Rama walked up to the sea shore and bowed. He then created a seat of grass (*kush*) on the sand and sat down on it. Then, he offered prayers to the ocean.

Lakshmana looked upon Rama as his father and obeyed each and every word spoken by him. But this time, he did not agree with the manner Rama was handling the situation. But then, when Rama explained his reason for his actions; Lakshmana accepted it.

On the other side, when Vibhishana was leaving Lanka, Ravana had instructed Shardul and Shuk to keep an eye on him. The informants, disguised as monkeys, were privy to all that was happening on Rama's side of the ocean. They were happy to see Rama take Vibhishana on his side. They were so engrossed in watching the proceedings that they forgot about their guise and appeared in their real form. The monkeys noticed this, tied them up and took them to Sugriva. The King ordered them to be beaten mercilessly. The monkeys were eager to cut off their ears and nose.

However, the informants said, 'You are under the oath of your master Rama—that you shall not dismember us.' Lakshmana was amused with everything. He asked the monkeys to free the prisoners. He then told them to carry a message for Ravana and wrote it down on a sheet of parchment. The message read: 'Return Sita, or your end is near'.

The messengers bowed to Lakshmana and left. They reached Ravana's court. Ravana asked Shuk, 'Tell me, how is Vibhishana? He would have been ruling Lanka had he not run away. Now, he shall die. And how are the hermits and their army of monkeys?'

Shuk replied, 'Please listen to what I am saying, without getting angry. As soon as Vibhishana went to Rama and prayed for his protection, Rama crowned him as the King of Lanka. The monkeys saw us through our disguise and they beat us mercilessly. The ape (Hanuman) who had come here was the weakest. There were other apes mightier than him in the army. Dwividh, Mayand, Nal, Neel, Angad, Viktasey, Kehri, Kumud and Jamvant, are very powerful.'

Ravana did not like what he heard. He started abusing Rama, 'What is the worth of a person pleads like a child with the ocean?' The messenger at that moment gave Ravana the message sent by Lakshmana. Ravana asked his minister to read it out aloud. The gist of the letter said: 'Those opposed to Rama shall not find shelter or support even from the Tridev (Brahma, Vishnu and Mahesh). So, either accept Rama's protection, like Vibhishana, or get ready to fight and die.'

Shuk said, 'Lord, what is written is very true. Please return Janaki.' Ravana got furious and kicked Shuk. Shuk was a very learned sage, who had turned into a demon by the curse of Sage Agastya. So, he was not given to hot-headedness. Seeing Ravana fuming with rage, he calmly went to Rama, and after meeting him, went in to his ashram.

On the other side, it had been three days since Rama had begun pleading with the ocean to show him a way, but to no avail. Rama realized:

*vinay na maanat jaldhi jad, gaye teeni din beet!*
*Boley Rama sakop tab, bhay binu hoye na preet!*

(It has been three days since I have been requesting you to guide me, but nothing has happened. I think now, the time has come that I leave the softness behind, because without instilling fear, nothing works.)

Rama got furious. He asked Lakshmana to fetch his bow and arrows. 'I shall now dry up the ocean,' he said.

He said, 'Reasoning with a foolish man, talking about attachment with a deceiver, discussing a beneficial strategy with a miser, having a logical discussion with an emotional man, asking a greedy person to detach himself of all materialistic objects, expecting a person prone to anger to listen to a discourse on peace and goodwill and preaching God's devotion to a person who is intolerant—all these are like sowing seeds in the barren land and expecting a bumper crop.'

Lakshmana was very pleased to see Rama's reaction. He was the kind of person who was not given to soft treatment in situations.

Rama said, 'The Ocean is arrogant, and thus, did not listen to my pleas. Peace, pardon, simplicity and humility are the characteristics of saintly people. Using these with unruly, uncouth people will only bear such results. The ocean was taking advantage of *Saam niti* and not showing itself and I cannot be patient any longer. I shall dry it up with my arrows.'

Saying this Rama shot a powerful arrow into the ocean. The arrow, instilled with great powers, churned the ocean. Waves rose as high as the sky. This scared the aquatic animals too. There was chaos in the ocean. Even demons living in the netherland shook with fear.

Sagar got scared and appeared in front of Rama holding a platter full of offerings. He appeared in the guise of a hermit.

The ocean begged for forgiveness with folded hands. He said that the earth, water, fire, air and sky are all hard to understand by nature, they are lifeless (*jad*), their functions are also unreasonable. 'My Lord, it is you who has set our parameters and have instilled us with the nature we have,' he said.

The ocean further said, 'If I dry up because of your powers, my dignity will be undermined. Please advise me on what I should do. What is that you wish for? I shall do your bidding, but please do not do anything that is against the laws of nature.'

Rama said, 'O great one! My intention is to reach the other side of the ocean along with my army. So now, please tell me how to do this?'

The ocean said, 'You have two apes, Nal and Neel, in your army. They are the sons of Vishwakarma. When Vishwakarma was born on Earth as a monkey due to a curse, they were born to him. The two are blessed and have very special powers. Their touch, with your divinity, shall make stones and rocks, float on the water surface. I shall also provide all support to the best of my abilities. This way, you can construct a bridge over the sea and cross to the other side.'

Hearing what the ocean had advised, Rama turned towards his ministers and said, 'What is the point in delaying? Please make preparations for the construction of the bridge.'

Jamvant sent for Nal and Neel, and asked them to chant the Lord's name and start the construction of the bridge in his name. Jamvant instructed the bears and apes to fetch trees and boulders. Nal and Neel, chanting the name of the Lord, threw the trees and boulders into the ocean, and they began to float. The trees and rocks entwined with each other and formed a road-like structure.

When the army of apes and bears were busy with Nal and Neel throwing stones into the ocean, Rama also picked up a stone and threw it into the ocean. The rock went straight down to the bottom of the ocean. Rama was very embarrassed and wondered if anyone had seen him. He saw Hanuman looking at him. Rama looked away, unable to meet his gaze. Hanuman let out a laugh and said, 'Lord, this is what will happen if you leave someone. He will just drown.'

A tiny squirrel also was helping out Nal and Neel. It picked up tiny stones and passed them to Nal and Neel. Rama, who saw this, was moved by the squirrel's devotion. He lovingly caressed its back. It is believed that the three stripes on an Indian squirrel's back are the marks of Rama's fingers.

The bridge was coming up fast, which filled Rama with joy and satisfaction. It was completed in five days. The total length of the bridge was 100 leagues.

Rama said that the seashore was a very scenic place. 'I wish to consecrate it to Lord Shiva. So first, I shall offer my obeisance to Lord Shiva, and then start for the battle.'

Rama asked Hanuman to fetch a Shivling from Kailash. Sugriva called many priests to consecrate the Shivling.

This way, all the preparations for the battle were made. The bridge was constructed and the Shivling, too, was established. Now, crossing the bridge to reach Lanka was the next step.

Vibhishana secured the Lankan end by crossing over to the other side and ensuring that no demon could damage the bridge. Rama, Lakshmana, Angad and Hanuman led the rest of the army to Lanka.

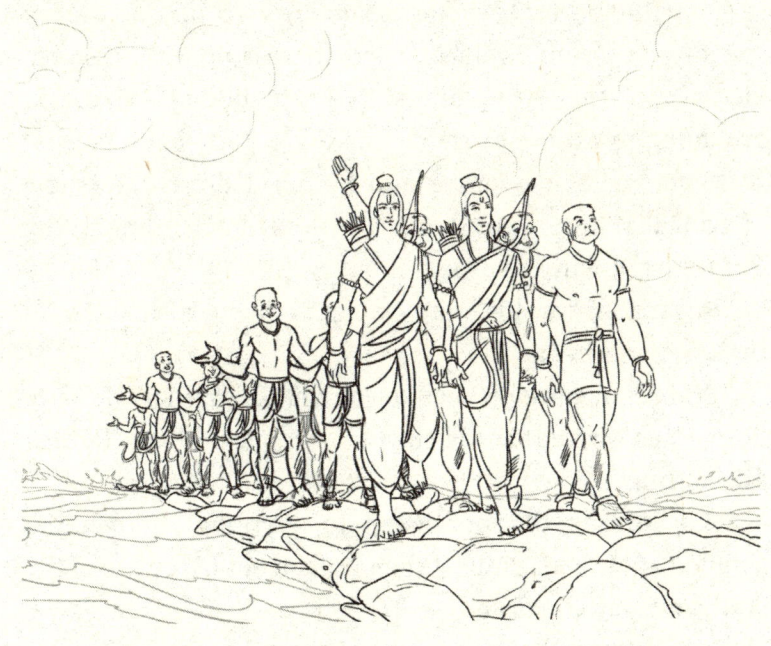

Mandodari was trying hard to persuade Ravana to return Sita to Rama and enter into a truce. She said, 'It is not in your favour to bear enmity with Rama. He has killed so many of your warriors. In fact, he has killed Vali too. He is Vishnu incarnate.'

Ravana consoled her and said, 'You are getting worried unnecessarily. There is no one in this world that can stand against my might. I have conquered Yam, Varun and Kuber. Why are you scared?'

Mandodari understood that Ravana's mind was in the grip of death and his arrogance had overshadowed truth. Ravana then entered his assembly and asked his ministers, 'How do we start the war?'

His ministers encouraged him and said, 'You need not fear anything. Monkeys and bears are our food.'

Ravana's son, Prahast, tried to reason with Ravana. He said, 'Father, your ministers are flatterers. What you are going to do is not right. There was only one ape that had come as a messenger and he burnt down the whole of Lanka. Where were these ministers at that time? Why did they not eat that single monkey?'

Ravana said to his son, 'Do not worry. We shall eat all the apes and bears.'

Prahast once again tried to convince his father. He said, 'Rama has arrived and is staying at mount Suhail. Return Sita to him.'

But Ravana did not listen to anything. In fact, he shouted at his son. Prahast then walked out of the assembly and went to his palace.

Rama reached Mount Suhail. He sat down and planned

the next step. This was a strategic location. So, he set up his camp there. Everybody started planning for the battle as per their responsibilities and positions.

Rama inspected Lanka by standing at the top of Mount Suhail. This peak of the Trikut mountain range was very high and seemed like it could touch the sky. Its sides and ground were covered with yellow flowers, giving it a golden hue. The mountain range spread over a 100 leagues. It seemed as if Ravana had got a golden stairway constructed to heaven.

After Prahast left for his palace, Ravana discussed the battle plan with his ministers. In the night, he went to the arena on the highest tip of Lanka and rested. The bards sang songs praising him.

Rama looked towards the vantage point where Ravana was resting. The area seemed to be well lit. He told Vibhishana, 'See, the clouds are gathering in the southern point; there is lightening too. It seems like it is going to rain.'

Vibhishana said, 'My Lord, this is not the rain, clouds or lightening. That is Ravana's palace and that place is Ravana's arena. He has a *chhatra* (umbrella) of artificial clouds. The lightening is actually the light reflected from Mandodari's earrings and the thundering is the sound of the percussion instruments (drum) that Ravana is listening to. Ravana is an accomplished musician too.' Rama interpreted this as Ravana's ego.

Rama shot an arrow which toppled Ravana's chhatra and Mandodari's earrings. Everyone seated in Ravana's assembly got scared and took it as a bad omen. They said that just by shooting one arrow, if Rama was able to topple Ravana's crown-umbrella, it should be taken as a serious warning. Therefore, Ravana should call for a truce with Rama. Ravana laughed it off. He said he had acquired boons from Lord Shiva by severing his heads and offering them to the Lord. So, this small incident should be taken as a blessing, not a bad omen. Then, all his ministers and courtiers went back to their homes.

But Mandodari was very worried. She tried to reason with Ravana again. 'Please understand the might of Rama, please return Sita.' She also said, 'When King Janaka had organized Sita's swayamvar, you were also there. Didn't Rama break the bow and marry Sita? Why did you not act at that time? Why did you not challenge Rama and conquer him there? He has blinded Jayant in one eye; you saw what Shurpanakha had to bear. Khar, Dushan and Kabandh were killed, but you still did not want to see what was in front of you. Even Marich recognized Rama. He also tried to dissuade you, but you did not listen to him. Tara had the power to see the future. She was aware of the outcome of Vali's war with Rama. That's why she had tried to stop him, but Vali did not listen to her. The result, you know very well! His messenger, Hanuman, shook you like a lion in a herd of elephants! You have already lost two sons.'

Mandodari further told Ravana, 'He has built a bridge. Even then, you are turning a blind eye to the events around you. You are also not trying to understand me, despite my best efforts. Now, I can see where you are headed.'

Ravana got irritated with Mandodari's nagging. He cut

short and said, 'Women always have their eight impious characteristics engrained in them!'

Mandodari said, 'Rama is Lord Vishnu incarnate. Please leave your animosity and stubbornness, and extend a hand of friendship so that I can enjoy a married life much longer and will not have to spend the rest of my life as a widow.'

Ravana did not pay any heed to it.

# The Battle of Lanka I

Ravana, with his ministers, went to the top of a mountain to take a look at Rama's army. His two ministers Shuk and Sharan informed him about the mighty apes and bears in Rama's army. They told him about their birth, characteristics, appearances and personalities, one by one.

They said in unison, 'O King! Look at this group of apes. The two mighty ones in the group are Nal and Neel. They are the sons of Vishwakarma. They had helped Rama in building the bridge over the ocean. The other ape, who has a golden hue, is Angad, son of Vali and Tara. The camp near Lanka is headed by the commander Dhoomketu, Jamvanta is Dhoomketu's brother. The yellow apes you see are 240 million in number. Their commander is a friend of Indra and Sugriva. He is the King of the apes, Kesri, and Hanuman's father. The other one is Sushen. Tara, wife of Vali, is his daughter. The one with an orangeish-red hue (*gerua*) and yellow eyes is Hanuman. He is the one who had set Lanka on fire. Surya is his guru. As a child, he had swallowed the sun and the whole world was engulfed in darkness. The two handsome princes are Shri Rama and his brother, Lakshmana. With them is Vibhishana, who knows all of our secrets.'

Ravana got irritated by the praise of his opponents, and he ordered his ministers to leave.

A demon, Shardul, infiltrated Rama's army and spied upon the soldiers to know about their preparations. On his return, he informed Ravana that it is difficult—or rather impossible—to gather any vital information about Rama's army. Now, it was his choice to either return Sita to Rama or face him on the battlefield.

Ravana, for the first time, became a bit wary. He called his important ministers for a secret meeting and tried to chalk out a plan, but failed. Ravana returned to his palace. He summoned the demon Vidyujivha, the master of illusions. He told him that he and Vidyutjihva would confuse Sita with their illusionary powers. So he ordered him to create Rama's head and a huge bow and arrow. Vidyutjihva did that and Ravana was very pleased with the creation. He took the bow and went to Sita, who was sitting sadly in the Ashok Vatika.

Ravana showed Sita the bow and said, 'The husband on whom you depended so much and refused to accept me for, has been killed on the battlefield and I have brought his head as evidence. Now, you only have the choice to accept me as your husband. Listen to how your husband was killed. He was camping with his army on the northern shore, it was past midnight and they were all in deep sleep. Under the command of Prahast my soldiers attacked and destroyed them. Prahast, cut off Rama's head and Sugriva's neck. He struck Hanuman on the chin and killed him. Lakshmana ran away from the battlefield.'

Thus, to convince Sita, Ravana took the names of all the important warriors of Rama's army and told her how they met their fate. He then ordered one of his demons to call Vidyutjihva. 'Go and call Vidyutjihva.' He asked him to show Sita the severed head of Rama so that she could have a last look at her slain husband. Vidyutjihva then placed Rama's illusionary head and vanished from the scene.

Ravana said, 'Look, this is Tribhuvan (three loks), the famous bow of Rama, which Prahast has brought here after killing Rama. Now you are in my control. Your saviour, Rama, is dead.'

Sita looked at the severed head, started crying and fainted. On regaining consciousness, she began to grieve and said, 'My Lord, you had been foretold a long life by the astrologers. How could you die so soon? You were an expert in the arts of warfare and use of weapons. So how did you die? Were you so deep asleep that during your slumber, the enemy could have overpowered you? How could you meet such a miserable end?'

She then said to Ravana, 'Either you kill me right now, or permit me to lay down my life along with my husband on his pyre. I want to see the rest of his body, please take me there.'

At that moment a soldier walked up to Ravana and said that Commander Prahast wanted to talk to him on an urgent matter. Ravana immediately left and as soon as he left the place, the bow and the head also vanished.

After Ravana left, Sarma, another demoness, who looked after Sita as her friend, came and said, 'I overheard your conversation with Ravana. I also know why he left in a hurry. Rama is invincible and his army of apes is also formidable. Rama is well-adept in the art of warfare. He is not dead. He cannot die so easily. Ravana is an illusionist and the head and bow were a creation of his powers. Your days of turmoil are over. Rama will very soon come and take you away from here after killing Ravana.'

Meanwhile on Suhail Hill, Vibhishana was updating Rama on the battle preparations on Ravana's side. He said, 'Prahast is guarding the eastern gate and Indrajeet is guarding the western gate. Ravana, along with Shuk and Saaran, are on the northern gates. Now, you can plan accordingly to defeat Ravana.'

Rama replied, 'Neel, you shall attack the eastern gate and tackle Prahast; Angad shall engage the soldiers of Mahaparshav and Mahodar at the southern gate. Lakshmana and I shall take on the northern gate where Ravana stands, and Sugriva, Jamvant and Vibhishana shall infiltrate and attack the city's centre. No ape shall take on a human form in this battle. This shall be our tactic to differentiate our army from theirs. Only the seven of us—I, Lakshmana, Vibhishana and his four ministers—shall remain in human form.'

Vibhishana once again went to Ravana and tried for the last time to convince him to return Sita. He said, 'Rama is invincible and it would be best for you to return Sita and seek forgiveness.'

He tried to explain to Ravana that a king has seven vices that lead to his downfall. They are—(1) Speech, (2) Harshness of Punishment, (3) Squandering of wealth, (4) Intoxication, (5) Lust (6) Hunting and (7) Gambling. Ravana also had them. But he did not pay any heed to them.

Rama addressed Jamvant, 'Tell us from your experience, how we should now proceed?'

Jamvant replied, 'We should send a message to Ravana for the last time to return Sita without engaging in a war. If he refuses, we shall fight.'

Rama then called Angad and asked him to convey the message to Ravana. He went to Ravana's court as Rama's emissary.

On his way, Angad met Ravana's son. He tried to stop Angad, but Angad killed him. Finally, Angad reached Ravana's court. A long argument ensued between the two.

Ravana said, 'Who are you?'

'I am the son of Vali and the messenger of Lord Rama. You were my father's friend, which is why I have come to try and save you. You are the grandson of Sage Pulastya. You have been a devotee of Lord Shiva and Lord Brahma. You have also conquered Indra and now, since you are drunk on power and lust, you have abducted Sita. Return Sita and ask for the Lord's forgiveness; he shall forgive you. Otherwise, it will not be good for you,' Angad said.

Ravana said, 'Yes, I do know a Vali, but how come you have come to me as a messenger of a hermit?'

Angad said, 'O Ravana! If I am a clan-destroyer, what are you, a clan-nurturer? Such words do not suit you. These words would not even suit someone who is deaf and dumb. You have ten heads, twenty eyes and twenty ears.'

Ravana said, 'I am aware of the principles of diplomacy, and that is precisely why I am listening to your harsh words.'

Angad said, 'I am aware of your patience and faith in

religion. You have abducted a woman who does not belong to you. A messenger is always protected from any harm, but what you did with a messenger is well known. I can see for myself that what I heard from Hanuman is true.'

Ravana fumed and asked, 'Who, in your army, is capable of fighting me? Rama is sad for being separated from his wife. Lakshmana is sad because his brother is upset. Jamvant is old and feeble. Vibhishana is a coward; Nal and Neel are artists, and they have no knack for a pitched battle. There is only one—Hanuman, the one who set my city on fire.'

Angad replied, 'He is not a warrior. He is a messenger. One who moves fast and travels long distances cannot be a warrior. We had sent him as a spy to gather information about you and your preparations for the battle. Did he really burn your city down? He was prohibited from any such activity. Maybe, that's why he has not gone back to Sugriva, due to the fear of being reprimanded. He is still hiding somewhere.'

Ravana said, 'What is wrong with you? Why have you come as the messenger of your father's murderer?'

Angad replied, 'Yes, he destroyed my father and now he will destroy you. You don't seem to know Vali's softer side and his charitable disposition. Which Ravana are you? I am unable to recognize you! I have heard of three Ravanas. Now you must listen to who they are—there is one who had ventured into the netherworld to hunt Bali and waged a war. The children there had tied him to a horses' stable and it was Bali who had freed him. The second Ravana was the one caught by Sahastrabahu, who thought Ravana to be an exotic creature and wanted to put him on display. He was saved by Sage Pulastya. The third Ravana was the one whom my father for ages held captive. He had gripped him so tightly that the Ravana was unable to move. Tell me, which one of these is you?'

Ravana replied, 'I am the Ravana whose antics are well-known in Mount Kailash and whose valour even Lord Shiva acknowledges. I have worshipped him and have offered my severed heads to him.

'Rama has no qualities of a ruler or a king. So, instead of being offered the post of crown prince, he was exiled,' Ravana further said.

Angad got offended and slammed his fist on the ground. The earth shook and a few of Ravana's courtiers fell down, while others ran away. Ravana too nearly lost his balance. His ten crowns fell off their heads. Ravana picked up a few and put them back on his heads. Angad picked up four and flung them towards Rama's camp.

Angad then slammed his foot on the ground and challenged the people present in the court to lift his foot off the ground. He vowed that Rama shall return without waging a battle, if anyone is able to do so.

Ravana's ministers tried to lift his foot but failed. Ravana was furious. He then got up himself and marched towards Angad. As he bent down to hold Angad's foot, Angad stopped him and said, 'Please do not touch my feet. Instead, you can touch Lord Rama's feet and as a result he will rid you of all your troubles. Ravana got embarrassed and he took his seat. Angad returned to Rama.

After Angad's departure, Mandodari again requested

Ravana to return Sita and extend a hand of friendship to Rama, but an arrogant Ravana mocked and ridiculed his wife.

When Angad returned, Rama asked him why he threw Ravana's crowns at him. Angad said, 'Lord, they were not just four crowns, they were, in fact, the four weapons of a king. According to the Vedas, speech, bribery, punishment and secrets are the four characteristics that are used to win over a person. I do not want Ravana to be victorious in future. So, I sent them to you.'

Rama wanted to test Angad's intelligence and now he was pleased. He then called everyone to his side and discussed the plan for the battle.

Rama's army attacked the four gates of Lanka. The apes and the bears hurled large boulders and rocks at the demons. Encouraged by Rama's love and affection, they waged such a fierce battle that the demons ran away from the battlefield to Ravana for help. Ravana got very angry. He ordered them to go back and fight. He warned them that if he found anyone running away from the battlefield, he himself would kill them. The demons thought that if they had to die, they would rather fight and die on the battlefield. So, they all went back to the battlefield, where Meghnad was fighting.

As a result, the apes started losing and called Hanuman for help. Hanuman rushed towards Meghnad with a huge rock and smashed his chariot. He then kicked Meghnad. Unable to bear the blow, Meghnad fainted. His charioteer managed to get him to a safe place away from the battle ground. The apes climbed atop the palace. After catching hold of the demons they dragged them and hurled them down. Angad and Hanuman climbed atop the fortress. They fought with the demons till sunset and went back to their camps.

But the sun hadn't actually set yet. This was an illusion by the demons. When they saw that Meghnad had fainted and was being carried off the field, they resorted to trickery and created an illusion of the sun setting. Scared of the darkness, the apes returned to their camps. Rama could see through the trick, and he shot off an *agni baan* (fire arrow), which illuminated the sky. The apes returned for a second round of battle.

Before the war began, everyone tried to persuade Ravana to end the battle, but failed. Even now no one was willing to continue with it. They knew that the results would be disastrous. One of the ministers was a pupil of Sage Pulastya, named Malyavan. He was also Ravana's cousin grandfather. He too had tried to deter Ravana from going to battle after Hanuman had set Lanka on fire. Again, with the onset of the battle, he had counselled Ravana to return Sita, but Ravan was too arrogant to listen to any of this.

Ravana had told Malyavan, 'Had you not grown old, I would have slain you for such advice.'

The next day, Meghnad returned to the battlefield. A fierce battle was fought and the apes got scared. Hanuman rushed towards Meghnad with a huge rock and hurled it at his chariot. The rock smashed chariot and the charioteer was killed. Meghnad, with his illusionary powers, flew away and vanished.

Meghnad then was visible everywhere. Rama shot an

arrow and put an end to the illusion. Then, Meghnad had to fight the battle with his real self.

Lakshmana came forward and engaged Meghnad in a battle. With the volley of arrows shot by Lakshmana, Meghnad got scared. In return, Meghnad shot many arrows with special powers but Lakshmana was able to ward them off effortlessly. Finally, Meghnad shot the *Shakti baan* (Power arrow), which struck Lakshmana in the chest. Lakshmana fell to the ground and was unconscious. Hanuman rushed to Lakshmana's help and carried him off the battlefield.

The battle lasted till the evening. Hanuman went directly to Rama and told him about Lakshmana. Hanuman said, 'Lord, during the fight between the two, Meghnad shot Lakshmana with the Shakti Baan and Lakshmana fell to the ground. He has been unconscious since then.'

Rama got worried and went to see Lakshmana. He began to cry. He said, 'Get up, Lakshmana! I will not be able to tell mother Sumitra that I have failed to protect my brother. To bear the loss of one's own brother is the most difficult thing to do.'

> *Vishwa may sab mil jaye, mil jaye mahipat ki thakurai,*
> *Kosh milay, vyapar miley, parivar miley, mil jaye lugai,*
> *Yeh sab vastu mahan, sulabh par durlab ek sahodar bhai.*
>
> (The ownership of a kingdom, treasures, business, family and wife—these things are great. But these can be acquired easily, or we can live without them.

However, a brother's love is higher than everything, and cannot be obtained under any circumstances if you don't already have it.)

'Because of your love for me, you left your parents. You stayed in the forest bearing all sorts of weather. Now, even after seeing me so restless, you are not waking up. Where has your love and affection for me gone now? Had I known that coming into the forest would separate me from my brother, I would not have obeyed my father. Please wake up.'

When Rama was mourning, Jamvant pondered over this issue. He suggested that instead of crying, they should try to find a way out of the crisis. If anything went wrong, they should first devise a means to set things right. Only after the situation has been brought under control, should they dissect the cause and reasons.

Vibhishana suggested that Sushen, who was a physician living in Lanka, might be of help. Hanuman was instructed to fetch Sushen. He found Sushen sleeping when he reached his house. Without wasting time to wake him up, Hanuman carried him, along with the bed, to Rama's camp. Sushen woke up and was dumbfounded. He said, 'I cannot treat Lakshmana, as he is Ravana's enemy and I am Ravana's subject. I shall be a traitor if I cure him.'

Hanuman was a diplomat to the core. He used all the techniques to convince Sushen to agree. He used the tactics of the Shastras—Saam, Daam, Dand and Bhed. He reminded Sushen of his responsibility as a physician and said, It should not matter who the person is, what time it is and what the circumstances are. He should just follow his professional ethics and treat the patient.' Sushen realised his duties and agreed to treat Lakshmana.

Sushen said, 'He needs the Sanjeevani Booti, which will act as an antidote for the Shakti Baan. You will find it in the north-eastern region of India. Arrangements should be made to fetch it at the earliest. If Lakshmana stays unconscious for too long, it will be impossible to revive him. Therefore, the herb has to be brought before sunrise.'

The next problem was who would get this medicinal plant in such a short time. Everyone looked at Hanuman at once, and so did Rama. Hanuman agreed, but expressed his doubts about recognizing the herb.

Sushen told Hanuman, 'It is easy to identify the herb, as it glows in the dark.' Hanuman bade farewell to everyone and promised to be back soon with the herb.

When Hanuman was on his way to fetch the herb from the Himalayas, Ravana conspired with the demon Kaalnemi to stop Hanuman.

Kaalnemi created a big garden with his illusionary powers. While Hanuman was going through the garden he became thirsty. He decided to settle in the garden to quench his thirst. He came across a lady sage. She told Hanuman, 'I am aware of the battle between Rama and Ravana and I am also confident that Rama will be victorious.'

She told Hanuman to freshen up, and she would then tell him a way to win the battle. He went to the pond to take a bath, where he was attacked by an alligator. The alligator gripped Hanuman's foot. Hanuman knocked off the alligator with a strong jerk, and it transformed into its original form of a Yakshini. She had been freed from a curse after being kicked by Hanuman. She flew away into the sky, but before flying away, she told Hanuman, 'The lady sage is a demoness in the guise of a sage and she wants to hurt you. You should be careful.'

When Hanuman returned from his bath, the disguised sage said, 'Come I shall now tell you how you could win the battle.'

Hanuman said, 'I do not need to know anything from you, instead let me tell you something.' He sprang into action and killed her. As soon as she died, the illusionary garden disappeared.

Hanuman transformed himself into his original huge self and set off in the north-east direction in search of the herb. After some time, Hanuman reached the hills of Dronagiri. It was covered with greenery. Due to heavy rains in the region, the plants had a fresh feel to them.

In Meghalaya and Assam, the moisture content in the air is very high, while glow-worms abound. It looked like stars had descended from the sky. Hanuman was confused between the twinkling of the glow-worms and the glowing herbs. He could not differentiate between the two, so he lifted the entire mountain and set off towards the camp.

When Hanuman was on his way back, he crossed over Ayodhya. Seeing a huge figure carrying a mountain, Bharata shot an arrow which struck him. Hanuman fell to the ground and cried, 'hey Rama'. Hearing Rama's name, Bharata rushed towards Hanuman. Bharata said: 'I thought it was a demon carrying the huge hill to crush Rama's army, but you seem to be a devotee of Rama. Please tell me about yourself.'

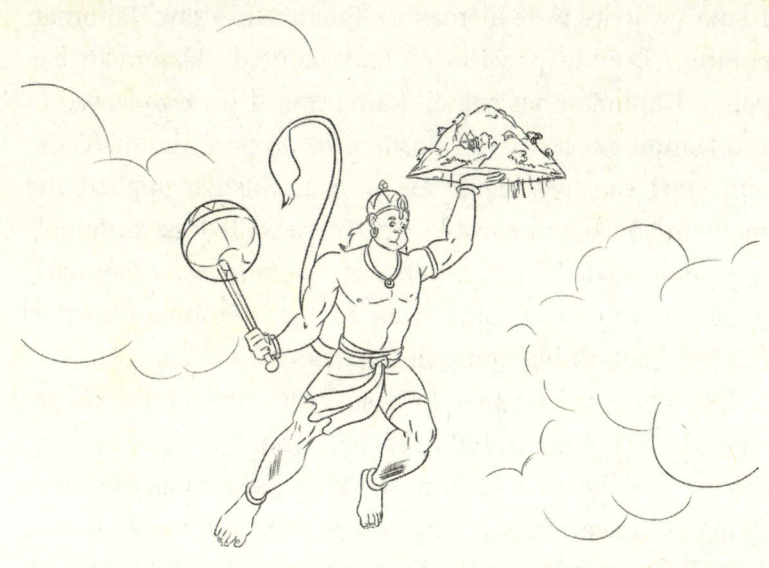

Hanuman said, 'I am Hanuman, a devotee and servant of Lord Rama. Meghnad has struck Lakshmana with the Shakti Baan. He is grievously wounded and unconscious. If I don't reach with this herb on time, Lakshmana will not be able to survive. I have to take this herb to him at the earliest.'

Bharata said, 'Okay. Please sit on my arrow and I shall send you to Lanka in no time.'

Hanuman was doubtful if the arrow would be able to bear the weight of the mountain and him, but he did not let the concerns show on his face. He told Bharata with folded hands, 'Please do not worry. I shall reach Lanka in time.'

To which Bharata replied, 'Okay, Do as you feel right.'

Hanuman was late and with every passing minute

*The Battle of Lanka I*

Rama's worries were increasing. Finally, they saw Hanuman coming. They leapt with joy and shouted, 'Hanuman has come, Hanuman has come!' Rama was also very pleased to see Hanuman. He asked Sushen, to prepare the medicine and start the treatment. As soon as Sushen applied the medicine, Lakshmana woke up. Tears welled up in Rama's eyes and trickled down his cheeks. Everyone was overjoyed to see Lakshmana come back to life. Hanuman carried Sushen back to his home in Lanka.

Ravana realised that he was losing the battle. So he went to wake up Kumbhakarna, who had been asleep during all these happenings. When Kumbhakarna was doing penance with Ravana and Vibhishana in the forest, Lord Brahma had granted Kumbhakarna the Nidrasan—he would sleep for six months and remain awake for just one day. Ravana woke him up and updated him with all that had been happening.

Kumbhakarna said, 'Brother, what you are doing is totally wrong. Do not challenge Rama. Return Sita and request Rama to forgive you.'

Ravana got irritated and rebuked Kumbhakarna. He said, 'I woke you up to help me, not to sermonize me. Tell me, will you help me or not? I have already lost quite a few warriors, along with Durmukh and Atikaye.'

Kumbhakarna said, 'I was just trying to tell you what is right, but you are my elder brother and I respect you. I shall definitely come to your rescue and obey you in toto.'

He then said, 'You stay back. I shall go alone, and come back only after slaying both Rama and Lakshmana.' Mahodar, one of Ravana's commanders, said,

'Kumbhakarna, you are talking like a petty soldier. Our king is also aware of what's right and wrong. He is not a child who knows nothing. The demons that were defeated by Rama in Janastana are still in awe and fear of his might. Our entire army is not sufficient to challenge him, and you are claiming that you alone shall slay both of them?'

Mahodar then turned to Ravana and said, 'You have got Sita in your custody. Now what are you waiting for? I have an idea: 'Announce that five of your warriors—Dwivid, Mayant, Mahodar, Kumbhakarna—are going to kill Rama. We shall go to the battle field and engaged in a fierce battle. If we are victorious, Sita is ours. On the other hand, if we lose the battle, we shall come to Sita and announce that Rama and Lakshmana are no more as we have eaten them. You shall then sit atop an elephant and announce the death of Rama and Lakshmana. With this, Sita will be heart-broken. She shall ultimately surrender to you, realising that there is no other choice.'

Kumbhakarna rebuked Mahodar for this silly plan and said to Ravana, 'Don't you worry, my brother. I shall fight Rama and Lakshmana on your behalf and win the battle for you.'

Since Kumbhakarna had woken up after a long sleep, he was miserably hungry, so he first had his meals—which comprised of a number of buffaloes and other small animals—before going to battle. In the battle field, he first met Vibhishana, who said with folded hands, 'Excuse me, brother, but I am supporting Lord Rama in the battle against Ravana.'

Kumbhakarna said, 'You are fortunate to be on his side.

I do not have a choice, despite my conviction that Ravana is wrong. I am morally bound to fight for him.'

Kumbhakarna created chaos in the battlefield, which resulted in heavy causalities. To counter his attack, Hanuman delivered a strong blow to his chest and Kumbhakarna stumbled. He fiercely attacked Hanuman, Nal, Neel, Angad and Sugriva and rendered them unconscious. He gripped Sugriva under his arm just like Vali had gripped Ravana. Sugriva slipped out of Kumbhakarna's grip and clawed at Kumbhakarna's nose and ears and tore them off. Kumbhakarna picked Sugriva up and slammed him onto the ground.

Kumbhakarna fought fiercely and the monkeys were scared. Then, Rama stepped in and challenged Kumbhakarna. Kumbhakarna picked up a hill and flung it at Rama. Rama stopped it midway with the help of an arrow. Finally, Rama shot arrows and killed him by cutting off his hands and head.

The next day, Meghnad entered the battlefield on a special chariot. He fought with his all might and created havoc in Rama's army.

Angad then challenged Meghnad and killed his horses and the charioteer. Meghnad, with his magical powers, vanished from the scene. Rama sent ten valiant commanders, comprising the two sons of Sushen along with Angad, Neel, Sharabh, Dwividh, Hanuman, Bhanuprasth, Rishab and Rishab Skand, to locate Meghnad. They looked for Meghnad in the sky, earth, and everywhere, but he was not to be found.

Indrajeet (another name for Meghnad) had been

blessed by Lord Brahma to become invisible at will. As such, whenever the odds were against him and he was low on energy, he used this trick to regain his strength and composure. In his invisible state, he rained arrows on his opponents. He struck Rama and Lakshmana with the deadly Naagpaash arrow (serpent-shaped arrow). It bound Rama and Lakshmana under its hypnotic spell (Moh Bandhan). The army of monkeys, seeing Rama and Lakshmana under the spell of the Naagpash got worried and demoralized. Eight commanders of Rama's army tried to defeat Meghnad and free Rama and Lakshmana, but failed. Meghnad gloated over his success, thinking he was still invisible and even Indra could not harm him. 'Rama and Lakshmana can also not trace me,' he thought.

The ten commanders who had been sent to locate Meghnad failed. However, Vibhishana could see Maghnad through his special powers. He told Sugriva, 'Calm down and detail monkeys as guards near the bodies of Rama and Lakshmana, till they regain consciousness. Meanwhile, I shall look after our army and try to lift their morale.'

Meghnad went back to the palace and told Ravana that he had killed Rama and Lakshmana. Ravana was overjoyed and embraced Meghnad. Meghnad then again returned to the battlefield in his invisible form, to instil terror in Rama's army.

Ravana, in the meantime, called the maids guarding Sita. He said to Trijita, 'Meghnad has killed Rama and Lakshmana. Take my Pushpak Viman and go to Sita. Bring her to the battle field. Show her, the two slain princes. She will be convinced that Rama's protection has ended and she herself will come to me.'

Trijita did as told. They took Sita to the battlefield. On seeing Rama's and Lakshmana's lifeless bodies, she was shocked. But Trijita consoled her by saying that her husband was not yet dead. Those who die do not have any glow on their visage. The Lord still had that glow intact. He was still alive.

Sita wished, 'May your words be true!' The Pushpak Viman then brought her back to Ashok Vatika.

Rama, due to his sheer determination, freed himself from the effects of the Naagpaash, but seeing Lakshmana also lying beside him said, 'Lakshmana had followed me to the jungle. Now, I shall follow him to the abode of Yamraaj (The Lord of Death).'

He asked Vibhishana, Jamvant and the others to end the war and go back to their homes.

Suddenly, Sugriva noticed a great commotion in the ranks of the army. He was first unable to understand what it was. Then, he saw Vibhishana coming. The apes had mistaken Vibhishana to be Meghnad and were running helter-skelter. Sugriva asked Jamvant to go and control them. Vibhishana was deeply grieved at the turn of events.

Vibhishana said to Sugriva: 'You should proceed to Kishkindha along with Rama and Lakshmana. I shall kill Ravana and bring Sita along. Meanwhile, Garud, the King of vultures, arrived. Seeing him, all the snakes slithered away. Garud wiped the faces of Rama and Lakshmana. They both regained consciousness immediately. Garud said: 'The snakes that have struck Rama and Lakshmana in the form of arrows are the sons of Kadru. They are extremely venomous. The demons tricked the sons with their powers and shot them at you in the form of arrows. Even the gods could not have helped you to wipe out their poisonous effect. As soon as I got the news, I came rushing.'

Finally, Garud flew back. Meanwhile, the contingent sent by Ravana under the command of Dhumraaksh, and Akampan, was killed by Hanuman, and the one under the command of Vajradanstra was killed by Angad.

After Akampan's death, Ravana went to Prahast and said, 'Now, the responsibility of this battle has fallen on our shoulders—Meghnad, you, Nikumbh and I. Therefore, now you lead the army and go to the battlefield.'

Prahast replied, 'I had told you in the beginning to settle the matter and return Sita to Rama, but you did not listen to me. Now, even though the situation has escalated to this level, I shall fight on your behalf because you have always taken care of me. I shall lead the army.' In the battlefield, Prahast was killed by Neel.

After Prahast's death, Ravana said that now he would join the fight himself. When Ravana appeared in the battlefield, Vibhishana said to Rama, 'Lord, this is Ravana.'

Rama stepped forward to challenge Ravana, but Lakshmana stopped him and said, 'Lord, I am capable of killing him; you stay here.'

Rama said, 'That's fine. You go and face him, but be careful. When Ravana fights with anger, not even the Gods can stop him. So you need to be aware of his weaknesses and use them in your favour. At the same time, you must hide your weaknesses so that he does not use them against you.'

Ravana was destroying Rama's army. Hanuman came forward but Ravana struck him with a hard blow. Hanuman stumbled, but controlled himself. Seeing Hanuman unsteady, Ravana engaged Neel. Neel jumped over the flag on his chariot and landed on Ravan's bow. Just then, an arrow struck Neel and he fell on the ground.

At that moment, Lakshmana came in front of Ravana and said, 'Do not boast about yourself. You can only abduct helpless women.' A fierce battle ensued between Ravana and Lakshmana. In the end, Ravana struck Lakshmana on his forehead with the divine arrow gifted by Lord Brahma, which was more powerful than death. Lakshmana's grip weakened on his bow but he did not lose control and cut off Ravana's bow-string. Lakshmana grievously wounded Ravana as well. Ravana then struck Lakshmana with the divine arrow of Lord Brahma, the Shakti. Seeing the Shakti come towards him, Lakshmana tried to counter it with three powerful arrows, but they failed to stop Shakti. It struck Lakshmana in his chest. Lakshmana was set aflame by the pain caused by the divine arrow. Ravana came near Lakshmana and tried to lift him, but the same Ravana who had the strength to lift the Himalayas with all the Gods—Mandrachal, Merugiri and the three worlds together, on it—could not lift Lakshmana.

Hanuman intervened and delivered a heavy blow to Ravana's chest. He staggered and fell. Hanuman lifted Lakshmana and took him to Lord Rama. After attending to his brother, Rama challenged Ravana. Hanuman said, 'Lord, please sit on my shoulders and fight.'

Rama then sat on Hanuman's shoulder and fought

Ravana. In the meantime, Lakshmana also regained consciousness. During the fight with Rama, Ravana's bow and arrow fell down.

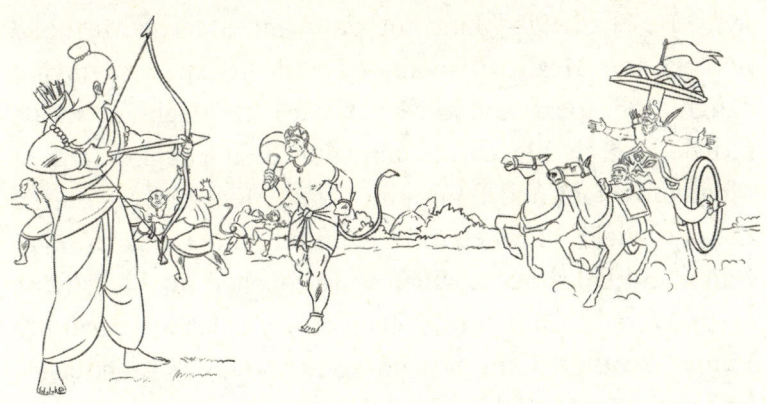

Rama then said, 'Ravana, I think it is enough for today. It seems like you are tired. Go back home. We shall continue our battle tomorrow.'

Ravana was moved by Rama's kind words and he thought to himself, 'When I had picked up Mount Kailash, Goddess Parvati had cursed me that a woman shall be the cause of my death. It looks like Parvati has been reincarnated as Sita and is out to destroy me. The curses of sages and holy men are not futile. Their curse seems to be turning true today.' Ravana left the battlefield. He is believed to have had seven curses on his head, which were the cause of his death.

Hanuman killed Ravana's second son, Trishira. Neel killed Mahodar and Rishabh killed Mahaparshav. Kumbhakarna's two sons, Kumbh and Nikumbh fought for five days. They were killed by Sugriva and Hanuman, respectively. Makraaksh, the son of Khar, was killed by Lakshmana.

The next day, Meghnad again came to the battlefield to fight. He challenged Jamvant. Jamvant attacked Meghnad fiercely and Meghnad retaliated with his spear. Jamvant caught the spear and threw it back at Meghnad which struck him in his chest. Jamvant then caught hold of Meghand's foot and flung him away. Meghnad re-entered the battlefield on his chariot. He fired numerous arrows at Rama and Lakshmana which were repelled by their divine arrow. Tired of shooting at each other, Lakshmana said to Rama, 'Brother, I am now going to shoot the Brahmastra and put an end to this.'

Rama stopped him and said, 'No, don't do that. It is not right to punish the whole universe for a single man's mistake. One who is in hiding and does not want to fight in the open, is not worthy of the Brahmastra. Let me try to kill him.'

Lakshmana said, 'He uses his ability to remain invisible. If he appears just for once, even our commanders will be able to kill him.'

Rama then said to Lakshmana, 'We shall now fire fast-moving arrows. They shall be able to locate Meghnad wherever he is hiding.' Meghand heard the conversation and fled the battlefield.

After the day's battle, Meghnad went back to Lanka. He went to the temple of Nikumbhla Devi to offer prayers and perform a yagn.

Vibhishana said to Rama, 'Meghnad is performing a

yagn at the Nikumbhla Devi's temple and if he is successful in completing it, he shall be come invincible, and even to the Gods. So, we should immediately leave for the temple and stop Meghnad from completing his yagn.' Rama advised Lakshmana to take his best warriors and go to the temple and destroy Meghnad's yagn. On reaching the temple, they found Meghnad performing the yagn. He was challenged and a fight between apes and demons broke out.

The apes devastated the holy fire and the yagn site. Clutching his hair, they pulled Meghnad away from the site. Meghnad took out his spear and attacked the apes. They rushed back to Lakshmana. The apes then engaged the other demons in a battle. Hanuman destroyed the demons' army and challenged Meghnad. After a duel between Meghnad and Hanuman, Lakshmana challenged Meghnad. Lakshmana killed Meghnad's charioteer and the apes killed Meghnad's horses.

Lakshmana fired the Varunastra at Meghnad and Meghnad fired the Rudrastra. Both their weapons nullified each other. Meghnad then fired the Agnayastra, which was negated by Lakshmana with his Suryastra. Meghnad then shot the Asurastra, which Lakshmana stopped with the Maheshwarastra. Finally, Lakshmana shot the Aendrastra, which separated Meghnad's head from his torso and killed him.

# The Battle of Lanka II

Ravana was furious when he heard about Meghnad's death and said, 'I shall destroy the root cause of this war! Meghnad had slayed an illusionary Sita; I shall kill the real Sita.'

One of the many tricks which had enfolded on the battlefield of Lanka was the killing of Sita, which was actually an illusion, to discourage Rama and his army. Ravana was referring to that incident. He drew his sword and rushed towards Ashok Vatika. Everyone tried to stop him on his way, but in vain.

At that moment, Suparshav, a minister in Ravana's court, stopped him and said that killing a woman was below his dignity as a valiant warrior. It would belittle his status. He advised Ravana to imagine the beauty of Sita, and goaded by her beauty, take revenge from Rama. He further said that that day was the last day of a waxing moon in the fortnight. 'Go to the battlefield tomorrow on the moonless night and get Sita after slaying Rama.' Ravana agreed to his minister's suggestions and went back to his palace.

When Lakshmana's arrow struck Meghnad, his head was separated from his torso. Hanuman picked up Meghnad's corpse and placed it at the main gate of Lanka, and he kept the severed head in front of Lord Rama.

Another tale associated with this says that when

Lakshmana's arrow struck Meghnad, his arm was cut off and it landed in Meghnad's palace in front of his wife Sulochana, daughter of Vasuki, the great serpent. Her maids said, 'It seems that the indestructible has been destroyed.'

Sulochan now feared the worst. She was aware that Rama and Ravana were fighting a fierce battle and her husband was also there. But she was confident that he had the strength to win over Lord Indra. That's why he was called Indrajeet. Therefore, it was not possible that her husband would be killed by a mere mortal. She also apprehended that this could be destiny. She rushed to the courtyard and looked at the arm. She recognized it as her husband's by the ruby bracelet that Meghnad used to wear.

Sulochna was curious to know who could do such a thing to her husband. She exclaimed, 'If I have been a woman of character, then this severed arm shall write the name down of my husband's slayer.'

The fingers of the severed arm spread out. One of the maids brought a piece of chalk and placed it in between the fingers of the arm. The arm then wrote a eulogy to his slayer: 'The person who can forgo food, sleep and bedding a woman for 100 thousand years is small in stature when compared to my slayer Lakshmana. He is invincible, indestructible and superior in all respects. He is the all-knowing and the all-loving. He creates, nurtures and destroys. He is one of the trios (Trimurti-Brahma, Vishnu and Mahesh). He is God and has taken birth as a human. Now, I am without a body and soul. So I cannot write his virtues. My head is with Lord Rama, and as a proof of my death, he has sent my arm to you.'

After learning the truth about Rama and Lakshmana, she mourned her husband's loss just like any other woman. She wailed and cried out loud in praise of her husband. She said, 'The hand that defeated Lord Indra has been severed from the brave man's body and is lying here in such a miserable condition.' She could not bear the loss of her husband. She pulled out all her ornaments and threw them on the ground. She fell on the ground and fainted.

Then, one of her maids approached her and said, 'Dear, do not grieve. You are intelligent and a woman of character and have been a devoted wife. Do what is in line with your status and character.'

Sulochna agreed with her friend and said, 'Yes, you are right.' She then called for a palanquin and sat in it with the severed arm. The citizens of the kingdom also followed the palanquin. The gate-keeper rushed and informed Ravana about everything. Ravana told the guard to bring Sulochana immediately to him.

Sulochana came to Ravana and said, 'The torso is still in the battlefield. The arm has been sent to me and the head is with Lord Raghunath (another name for Rama). This severed arm told me everything. If I am able to get the head, I shall die a peaceful death. Please try and get me the head of my husband.' Ravana was heart-broken. He slumped down, losing all hopes of continuing with this life, but still, his arrogance knew no bounds.

He said, 'Who is this warrior greater than me? I shall kill Rama, Lakshmana and Hanuman and get back my son's head. Till now, I have been dependent on my sons and brothers, but it is shameful that they have all been killed by mere men and apes. Now, I will fight. It is because of the sins committed in the previous lives that matters have gone out of hand. Otherwise, the apes stand no chance against these demons. But these apes have just vanquished mighty demons like mosquitoes.'

Sulochana said, 'Despite seeing the apes' strength and the destruction they have caused, you still consider them "mere" apes? Those who could kill Kumbhakarna, Mahodar and my husband, you think you can conquer them? This is foolishness! The only reason I'm not being harsher is that I do not want to disrespect you and become a sinner.'

Sulochna then went to Mandodari. She informed her of what had happened. Madodari became very sad. She said, 'My dear daughter, whatever Sage Narad had predicted has come true till now, and shall also be in the future. So, it is best that you perform Sati and reserve a place for yourself in heaven. Go to Rama and request for your husband's head. Do not hesitate. You have no place for modesty today. Bad times do not have any place for such attributes. He is a man who respects women; Rama is a man of principles and advocates that a man should have only one wife. Vibhishana is your father-in-law; Angad is like a son to me. Thus, there should be no fear in going to him.' Sulochana, agreeing with Mandodari's advice, went to Rama.

When she stood in front of Rama, Vibhishana introduced her to him. Sulochana stood with folded hands and said to Rama, 'Shree Rama, I have come to beg you for something.

*The Battle of Lanka II* ❦ 133

If you could give me my husband's head, I shall be a Sati and end my life in peace.'

She also told Rama about the severed arm. He said, 'If you want, I could revive him and he could rule over Lanka.'

Hearing this, the apes were taken aback. They were scared that if Lord Rama did bring back Meghnad, he would start the war all over again and Vibhishana's ascent to the throne would be cast into doubt.

Sulochna said, 'Lord, I do not wish for him to be alive again. He was feared by everyone in the world. It would not be proper if I beg for his life. It would be an insult to my husband. Now, I will follow only the right path of sati.'

Rama agreed with Sulochana. He asked Vibhishana to bring Meghnad's head. Vibhishana brought the head and gave it to Sulochana. She wiped the dust and grime off his face and looked at it sorrowfully.

Then, Sugriva said, 'How could an arm, severed from the body, be able to write? I will only believe this if this face could laugh. Otherwise, it is nothing but an illusion created by the demons.'

Rama stopped Sugriva and asked him not to be rude, but Sulochana asked for her husband's head to laugh.

She said, 'You are tired after the battle. Lakshmana's arrows made me a widow and now I have to bear insults because of you, in front of Rama! If I have been a true wife, you shall laugh! Laugh, so that your departure is enveloped in infinite fame and praise! My Lord, if I had known that you would meet such an end, I would have called for my father for help!'

Hearing such words from his wife, Megnad's let out

a throaty laughter. The apes and bears were taken aback.

In fact, it was actually Meghnad laughing at her innocence and naivety, as she was unaware that Lakshmana was Sheshnaag incarnate. After taking Meghnad's head, she requested Lord Rama to stop the war for the day at that very moment.

She then spoke to Vibhishana and said, 'The future of the clan is now in your hands. As you are the Kuldeepak or the scion of the Pulastya clan, may you rule Lanka for ages.' Vibhishana escorted Sulochana to her palanquin. She went to the battlefield to pick up the body of her husband. She then went to the confluence of the sea and the river. Ravana and Mandodari were waiting for her with the entire royal household. The pyre was decorated with incense, *agar* and sandalwood. Sulochana sat on it with her husband's body and the pyre was lit. Sulochana, as sati, holds a great significance in Hindu mythology.

Ravana and Mandodari mourned Meghnad's death. At midnight, Ravana called his son Ahiravana, who was also known as Mahiravan, with the Aakarshan Mantra. Ahiravan knew that his father was in distress, but he could not figure out the reason. He came to Ravana. Ravana told him the entire story, starting from Shurpanakha's incident, the death of Khar, Dushan, Maricha, Sita's abduction, the burning of Lanka, war with Rama and deaths of Kumbhakarna and Meghnad. Then, he said that he had called Ahiravana for help.

Ahiravan was the king of the Netherlands, where serpents lived. After listening to the whole story Ahiravan said, 'To help you, I will kidnap Rama and Lakshmana.

I will offer them as a sacrifice to the Goddess of the netherworld. When you see a light as bright as sunshine, you will know that I am carrying them away.'

After the battle ended for the day, Hanuman drew a circle with his tail and sat guard at the entrance of the camp. Ahiravan entered the battlefield. First, he hailed Rama in his heart and then disguised himself as Vibhishana. He approached Hanuman and said, 'I had gone for evening prayers. I have now come to meet Lord Rama. I want to offer my apologies to him, since I am late.'

He reached Rama's tent and offered salutations. He rendered everyone unconscious. He picked up Rama and Lakshmana and vanished. There was a bright light in the sky and Ravana knew that Ahiravan had got the work done. Ahiravan reached the kingdom with the princes.

When all the apes of Rama's army woke up and realised what had happened, they started searching for Rama and Lakshmana. Vibhishana, Sugriva and Jamvant were worried.

Hanuman said, 'Someone came in Vibhishana's disguise and said he was going to meet Lord Rama.' Vibhishana concluded: 'I am sure Ahiravan has abducted Lord Rama. Only Ahiravan can take my form so it must be his work. Now, we should send someone very powerful who can defeat Ahiravan.'

Jamvant said to Hanuman, 'The world swears on your might and power. Only you can get us out of this situation.' They reminded him of his powerful deeds like leaping across the ocean and retrieving the Sanjeevani Booti.

Hanuman said, 'You take care of the army. I will search

for Rama and Lakshmana and bring them back.'

Hanuman started his journey. On his way, he overheard a discussion between two vultures. They were saying that Ahiravan had taken Rama and Lakshmana to offer them as a sacrifice to their Goddess. 'We are fortunate enough to get human flesh to eat,' they said.

Hanuman went to Ahiravan's kingdom. Its gate was guarded by an ape, Makardhwaja. He told Hanuman, 'I am the son of Pawanputra.' He was as faithful to the Lord as Hanuman.

Hanuman asked him, 'I am unmarried. How do you claim to be my son?'

Makardhwaja said, 'During the Lankan inferno, I was conceived by a fish which had consumed your sweat.'

Hanuman said, 'Okay. Now tell me where Ahiravan has taken Lord Rama and what he intends to do with him?'

Makardhwaja said, 'I have heard that he is going to sacrifice them to his Goddess. I am telling you the truth, but cannot allow you to go there. I must perform my duty sincerely like my father.'

When Hanuman tried to enter the kingdom, a fierce duel began between them. Both were brave and powerful. So, there was no end to this. At last, Hanuman won over him and tied him with his own tail and moved ahead. Hanuman transformed into his miniscule self and entered the sacrificial site.

There was a statue of a goddess, a sacrificial alter, lots of animals, and pots brimming with blood and meats. Then, a lady gardener passed Hanuman with a basket full of flowers. Hanuman transformed himself into a fly and hid himself among the flowers. She offered those flowers along with Hanuman to the Goddess. Hanuman sat on the goddess and began to grow. The goddess, in submission, touched Hanuman and assimilated herself into the earth. Hanuman now stood in place of the goddess. Then Hanuman transformed himself into Panchmukhee Hanuman (five-faced Hanuman). It is believed that this was the place where the five-faced avatar of Hanuman gained prominence.

When the demons saw the five-faced Hanuman, they thought that their Goddess was very pleased and had appeared in a rare form. They began their prayers and offerings. Hanuman consumed all the goodies. Then Ahiravan brought Rama and Lakshmana to the sacrificial site and placed him in front of the goddess. All the demons were armed with swords, spears, bows and arrows.

The chief priest said that there were still three minutes until the auspicious time. Ahiravan told Rama that they should remember their dear ones. Rama and Lakshan looked at each other and smiled.

Everything is predestined. Ahiravan lifted his sword to kill Rama and Lakshmana. Hanuman sprang up with a loud roar. The demons thought that the goddess was unhappy with Ahiravan's deed of kidnapping Lord Rama. Hanuman picked up Rama and Lakshmana and put them on his shoulders. He snatched the sword of one of the demons and killed each one of them. In the end, he chopped off Ahiravan's head and put it into the sacrificial fire as poornahuti (the last offering). Hanuman, after killing Ahiravan and the demons, flew away. At the gate, he met Makardhwaja and blessed him to become the king of the netherworld. They left for the Lankan battlefield. Seeing Rama and Lakshmana, everybody was relieved and shouted slogans in praise of Rama, Lakshmana and Hanuman.

When Ravana heard of Ahiravan's death, he fainted. When he woke up, Mandodari tried to show him reasons to withdraw from the battle, but he was blinded by arrogance.

Infuriated with Ahiravan's death and Mandodari's constant sermonizing, Ravana started pacing up and down the chamber. One of his ministers, Sindoornaad, paid him a visit. He said, 'Why worry? You still have a son who is powerful.'

Ravana said, 'Now there is no warrior left in my clan.' Sindoornaad reminded him about his one son who was born during an inauspicious time (Mool Nakshatra). He was considered to bring bad luck to the family. On the same day and at the same time, seventy-two crore children had taken birth in Lanka. His Guru Shukracharya said that these children should be locked up in boxes and thrown into the sea. Somehow, all the boxes stuck to each other like a honeycomb. The boxes got entangled with the roots of a banyan tree. In due course, the roots of the banyan tree entered the boxes and the children inside them fed on the milk of the banyan tree.

Seven years passed by. They had grown up to become strong boys. They had travelled together to the confluence of River Ganga and the sea, where they met Sukracharya.

Sukracharya told them the story of their birth. They decided to stay back there and get educated. All of them became devotees of Lord Brahma. They performed penance for 1,000 years. Lord Brahma was pleased with them and offered them a boon.

Narantaka said, 'Please bless us with invincibility. No one ever should be able to defeat us.'

Lord Brahma said, 'So be it. But remember to never fight with Sugriva's son. He is your Guru Bhai (classmate). If you do so, you will die.'

After giving this boon to Narantaka, Brahma asked others what they desired.

They said, 'We wish to be victorious in the battle between gods and demons.'

Lord Brahma said, 'You shall be invincible to any living creature, barring apes and bears.'

Narantaka created a city named Bihvavalpur in the sky with the blessings of Lord Shiva. There, seventy-two crore homes of gold, studded with gems, were made for them.

There was a baby ape named Dadhibal. He stayed and studied with them. One day, in a fit of rage, their teacher admonished Dadhibal and cursed him that he would be responsible for his guru brother's death. Dadhibal maintained his self-respect and taking his teacher's leave, left the city. On Narad's advice, he became a devotee of Lord Shiva, Parvati and Rama. He went to Dhavalgiri Mountain, settled down and started to meditate. While Dadhibal was engrossed in meditation, Narantaka spent his time conquering kingdoms and became a powerful king.

Ravana called for a special messenger, Dhoomketu, who was also a minister also in Ravana's court. Ravana ordered him to fetch Narantaka. When Dhoomketu met

Narantaka, they exchanged pleasantries. Then, he conveyed Ravana's message to Narantaka. Narantaka immediately ordered his army to get ready to join his father. His wife Bindumati told him that she will accompany him to their in-laws' place. All of them reached Lanka. Narantaka met his father and Ravana gave him all the details about the war. Next day, in the battlefield, Narantaka was challenged by Hanuman and Lakshmana. Narantaka threw a spear at Lakshmana, but Jamvant caught hold the spear midway. Jamvant slammed Narantaka on the ground and then flung him away. Narantaka landed near Ravana.

The next day, Narantaka launched an aerial attack. A fierce battle ensued between the apes and demons, surrounding them with darkness. The apes got confused. At that time, Rama shot an arrow and the battlefield lit up.

The next day, Narantaka was challenged by Angad and Hanuman. Narantaka wounded them. Rama advised Lakshmana to take up the challenge. Lakshmana collapsed due to injuries. After a while, Lakshmana gained consciousness and returned to the fight.

In the evening, Narad came to Rama and said, 'Lord, you are omniscient. You know all. Even then, Brahma asked me to convey a message to you. You should send someone to bring Dadhibal, the son of Sugriva. Only he can kill Narantaka.'

Rama called Hanuman and asked him to bring Dadhibal from Dhavalgiri Mountain. Hanuman flew to Dhavalgiri. He conveyed Rama's message and Dadhibal agreed to accompany him to the battlefield, where Dadhibal met Rama, Sugriva and Angad.

The next day, Narantaka met his classmate Dadhibal on the battle field. Both were very happy to see each other after such a long time. They exchanged pleasantries. Dadhibal tried to convince Narantaka not to fight against Rama.

Narantaka said, 'You monkeys are cowards by nature, and befriend your enemies. This is not the tradition of demons.'

They started fighting each other. Narantaka flew to the sky with Dadhibal, but Dadhibal threw him back to the ground. Narantaka died on the spot. Dadhibal beheaded him and flung his body towards Ravana's palace. He brought the head to Rama.

Rama said, 'Keep the head safely. I am very pleased with your efforts. Now you may ask for a boon.'

Dadhibal said, 'I want to remain engrossed in your worship.' Rama said, 'So be it.'

Rama also gave him the kingdom of Bihvavalpur.

Narantaka's torso fell where Ravana was seated. He was overcome with grief. Mandodari suggested to Bindumati that she should go to Rama and request him to give her the head of her husband. Narantaka's wives—Bindumati and Chitralekha—went to Rama. He gave them the head of their husband and ordered Vibhishana, Angad and Hanuman to prepare a pyre. Both wives of Narantaka sat on the pyre and it was lit up.

Ravana had lost all his family members and warriors in the battle. Now there was no one left in his family and clan. So, he walked on to the battlefield himself.

When Rama stepped into the battlefield to fight Ravana,

Vibhishana said, 'Lord, Ravana is riding a chariot and you are on foot. You do not even have an armour. This battle is not being fought on equal terms. How will you fight him?'

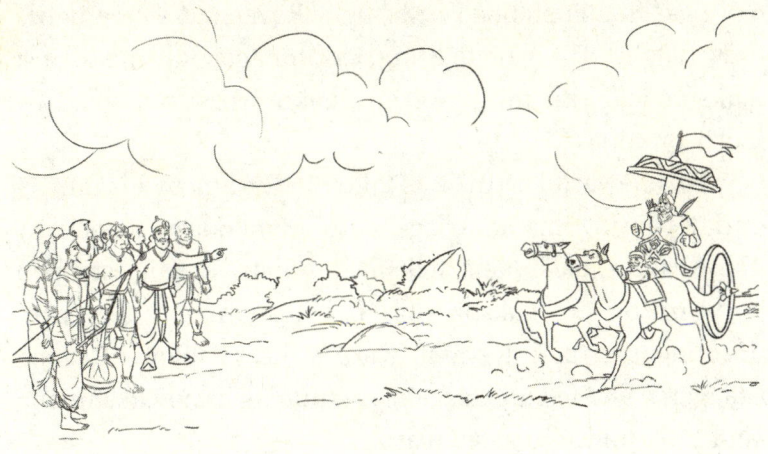

Rama said, 'Friend, my chariot has the wheels of valour and patience, the flag atop my chariot is of truth and humility, it is drawn by the horses of might, intelligence, character, control over senses (*indriya*) and welfare, and they are reined in by absolution, compassion and equality. The chants of the Lord are my charioteer and my shield is my detachment, my oneness. Satisfaction is my sword, charity my hacker, intelligence is my unbridled power and great knowledge and science is my bow, my quiver is my unwavering heart filled with arrows of principles, ideals, rules and ethics. Respect to the Brahmins and offering of prayers to a teacher are my armour. There is no other way to victory. When I am so well prepared, I do not think victory should be difficult.'

In the battle, the apes flung rocks and boulders at Ravana. Enraged, he started crushing them. They started to run around and shouted, 'save us, save us!'

Lakshmana stepped in to fight Ravana. A fierce battle was fought. Tired of fighting Lakshmana, Ravana struck Lakshmana with the powerful Shakti arrow sanctified by Lord Brahma.

This powerful arrow was gifted to Ravana by his father-in-law during his marriage with Mandodari. Struck by the Shakti, Lakshmana fell unconscious. Ravana stepped forward to lift Lakshmana, but Hanuman intervened. Hanuman struck Ravana with a heavy blow. Ravana staggered and fell unconscious. Hanuman lifted Lakshmana and took him to a safer place.

Ravana's charioteer took him away from the battlefield. On regaining consciousness, he became very angry. He rebuked the charioteer and said, 'Why have you brought me away from the battlefield? You have ruined my efforts and disgraced me. Have you been bribed by the enemies to do such a thing?'

The charioteer replied, 'It is not what you think, my Lord. You seemed tired and the horses too were exhausted. I feared the worst. So for your safety, I brought you away from the battlefield. A charioteer is supposed to have the intelligence to gauge a situation and circumstances and take appropriate actions at the right time.' Ravana agreed and said, 'Good, now let us go back to the battlefield again.'

Hanuman brought the unconscious Lakshmana to Rama. Rama said, 'Lakshmana, as you are the destroyer of death and the protector of gods, you must wake up!' Lakshmana woke up and went back to fight Ravana. This time, when Lakshmana attacked Ravana, he collapsed and his charioteer again took him away from the battlefield.

On the second day, Ravana fought throughout the day without a victory. In the evening, he thought of going to his temple. He prayed and offered a sacrifice to get God's blessings.

Vibhishana warned Rama and said, 'Ravana is performing the Ajay Yagn (the yagn for invincibility). You should not let him complete it. Destroy it.'

With Rama's permission, Angad, Hanuman and a few apes went to the temple and created havoc, dragging the women-folk out. Ravana lost his temper at the behaviour of the monkeys and got up to chase them away. In the meantime, the other monkeys destroyed the yagn.

The next morning, Ravana again went to the battlefield. This time, Lord Indra had lent his chariot and his charioteer, Matali, to Lord Rama, to face Ravana. Rama fought Ravana with his Shaang bow. There was a fierce battle between the two. Ravana resorted to trickery and created an illusion of Rama and Lakshmana everywhere on the battlefield. The monkeys got confused. Sensing it was a trick, Rama shot an arrow and the illusion was destroyed.

Ravana boasted about his capabilities and began to sing songs praising himself. Rama interrupted him and said that there are four kinds of plants and trees: 'The first type is that which bears only flowers, like the rose, etc. The second type is that which bears flowers and fruits, like the mango tree. The third type is that which bears only fruits, such as the jackfruit, and lastly, there is the type which neither bears flowers nor fruits. Similarly, men are also of four types—those who only talk but do nothing; those who talk and do what they say; then, those who only accomplish tasks but say nothing; and the fourth type, who neither accomplish the task nor talk about it. You belong to be the third variety of people—who just accomplish the task and do not talk about it. So just fight and stop bragging.' Ravana, in his anger, shot the Asurastra, and filled the sky with arrows. Rama shot an Agneyastra which burnt all the arrows in the sky.

Rama shot arrows at Ravana. Each arrow cut off one of his heads and arms. But no sooner were they severed, they were replaced by a new one. There was no end to the long drawn battle. The gods witnessed the battle from their abode in heaven. Sage Agastya also joined the audience. He advised Rama to chant the *'Aditya Hridye Strota'*. He also assured Rama that he shall be victorious and that he should not be disheartened. Rama, with a pure heart, chanted the strota and his charioteer reminded him to use the Bramhas—which Lord Brahma had gifted to Lord Indra.

Ravana attacked Rama with all sorts of weapons—*chakras* and *trishuls* (trident)—but Rama destroyed all of them. Ravana then fired at Vibhishana with three Shaktis together. Rama pushed Vibhishana aside and faced them himself. Rama felt slightly jolted but regained composure in no time. In the meantime, Vibhishana rushed towards Ravana and kicked him hard on the chest. Hanuman also joined Vibhishana and he broke Ravana's chariot and killed the horses and the charioteer.

Ravana then attacked Hanuman. Hanuman flew off to the sky. Ravana pulled him back by his tail and both started fighting. The other monkeys also joined the fight. Ravana then created an illusion where there were hundreds of Ravanas. The monkeys got confused. Rama again shot an arrow and the illusion was destroyed.

---

In the Ashok Vatika, Trijita narrated the proceedings of the battlefield to Sita and said, 'Despite being shot continuously by Rama's arrows, Ravana is still alive.' Sita got depressed and worried about what would happen next!

Trijita told Sita that one always dies when struck in the heart. Ravana should also die when he is struck in the heart. But Ravana had Sita in his heart. Therefore, if Rama shot an arrow at his heart, it would strike Sita too. In Sita's heart resided Rama, and in Rama's the whole world (fourteen Bhuwans). So, Rama would not strike Ravana with his arrows in his heart. He would cut off Ravana's heads and arms one after the other, and when Ravana lost his temper to the extent that he stopped thinking about Sita, Rama would strike his heart.

The battle for the day ended and the following day, another round of a fierce battle was fought between Rama and Ravana. Ravana tried all sorts of tricks and illusions, but no conclusive end was achieved. Ravana gave out a loud roar, as a result of which Lakshmana, Sugriva and many other apes fell unconscious.

Ravana again created hundreds of Hanumans around

Rama by his magical powers and Rama shot an arrow and destroyed the illusion again.

Then, Vibhishana told Rama that a pot of elixir had been brought from heaven and hidden in Ravana's navel. In fact, it was Vibhishana himself who had planted it there. So first, Rama should shoot an arrow and dry up the pot of elixir, only then could Ravana be killed.

Following Vibhishana's advice, Rama shot an arrow at Ravana's navel, as a result of which the pot of elixir dried up. Then, Rama continued to chop off Ravana's ten heads and twenty arms. This time, the heads and arms did not regrow, and Ravana fell to the ground, devastated and destroyed.

As Ravana fell, the war came to an end. Rama asked Lakshmana to go to Ravana. He said, 'Ravana is a learned scholar, an accomplished politician, a great musician, and adept in the art of diplomacy; go and learn them from him.'

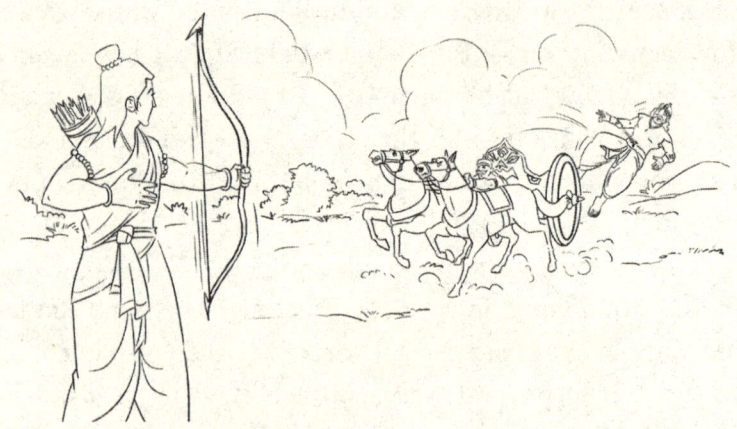

Lakshmana went to Ravana and said, 'I have come to you to gain knowledge. Please impart some wisdom to me.'

Ravana did not reply. Lakshmana repeated his request thrice, but Ravana still did not reply. He returned to Rama and said, 'I requested him thrice but he did not reply. Thus, I have come back.'

Rama asked Lakshmana, 'Where were you standing when you made the request? Were you near his feet or head?'

Lakshmana said that he was standing near the head. Rama said, 'Lakshmana, you did not follow the basic rules of a teacher-student relationship. When you went to him to gain knowledge, he had become your teacher. The enmity was left behind. A teacher has to be respected as per his status and position. Students should stand near their teacher's feet. Go back to him and follow my advice.'

Lakshmana went and stood by Ravana's feet and requested him to impart some knowledge. This time, Ravana opened his eyes, looked at Lakshmana and imparted to him the following three sermons.

1. Never put off today's work for tomorrow. I had planned to make the water of the ocean sweet but due to my laziness, I kept delaying the matter. Now see, I am leaving and the matter remains unaccomplished.
2. Never be dependent on anyone else. Undertake work which you feel that you can do by your own abilities and capabilities. I wanted to build a staircase of gold leading up to heaven. I was capable of completing it myself, but depended on Vishwakarma for this task. As a result, I am going to heaven without building the staircase.

3. Never underestimate anyone. When Lord Brahma refused to grant me the boon of immortality, I asked him to make me invincible against all creatures except humans and monkeys, as I thought myself to be much superior and powerful to them. But see, today, the same Ravana who had defeated the gods and yakshas is lying on the death bed wounded and incapacitated by a human and his army of monkeys!

Lakshmana, after learning these lessons from Ravana, left.

Ravana then asked Rama, 'Who has been victorious, you or me? Who is the braver of us, you or me? As long as I was alive, you could not enter Lanka, but see, you are alive and I am entering into your kingdom (heaven) with my whole family, and you shall not be able to stop me. I called all my family members from far and near and made sure that they were killed in the battle before me. My entire family has been killed by you and has attained a place in your abode. Now I, too, am going there.' Ravana then let goes off his soul.

Vibhishana was very sad after Ravana's death. He grieved, 'Brother, how many times did I try to show you the virtuous path, but you did not listen to me. Now see, what has come of you!'

Vibhishana also thought to himself:

*Ek lakh poot, sawa lakh nati! Ta Ravana ghar diya na bati!*

(This is the irony of fate! Ravana was blessed with a hundred thousand sons and a hundred and twenty-five thousand grandsons. But during his last moments, there was not a single man to offer him water or solace, or light a lamp, which is done after the death of a person.)

The women-folk of the house also started crying and wailing. Rama said to Vibhishana, 'Enmity lasts as long as the person lasts. Now that our task has been fulfilled, go and arrange for an appropriate cremation ceremony for Ravana. At present, he is worthy of your as well as my compassion and affection.'

Vibhishana performed the last rites of Ravana, and Rama asked Matali to take back Lord Indra's chariot. He also instructed Lakshmana to crown Vibhishana as the King of Lanka. Lakshmana did as was told.

Rama asked Hanuman to go to Sita and convey the good news of Ravana's death. Hanuman took Vibhishana's permission and went to Ashok Vatika and conveyed the news to her. Sita was spellbound with happiness.

Hanuman asked her, 'Why don't you say something?'

She said, 'I am very happy. I want to gift you something. You have given me such good news, but alas, at present, I do not have anything to offer you! There is actually nothing, which can be equated with the happiness that I have received from this news.' She also expressed her desire to meet Rama at the earliest. Hanuman came back to Rama and conveyed Sita's desire. Rama asked Hanuman and Vibhishana to go and bring Sita. Rama instructed Hanuman not to bring Sita in a palanquin, but ask her to walk all the way down, so that every soldier, every monkey

*The Battle of Lanka II* ॐ 151

and every bear sees her.

Hanuman and Vibhishana went to Sita and told her, 'Rama has called for you.'

Trijita, dressed Sita and sent her to Lord Rama along with Hanuman and Vibhishana. After Sita reached the battlefield, Vibhishana ordered the soldiers, 'Now that you have seen Mother Sita, please go back and leave her alone.'

Rama then once again said, 'No, Sita does not require any seclusion, nor a veil or distance.' Sita then stepped in front of Rama and he continued, 'I killed Ravana because he had challenged my prowess and self-respect. But you have been in his custody for such a long period! He had lifted you in his lap, touched you to place you on his *rath* (Pushpak Viman) at Panchwati. Therefore, you are no longer pure. I cannot accept you, as you are!'

Sita understood why Rama did not ask for privacy. He wanted everyone to listen to what he had to say!

Rama continued his criticism of Sita and said many harsh words. He went to the extent of demanding Sita to undertake the Agni Pareeksha (a test by fire or trial by fire) to prove her chastity. Sita was hurt listening to such harsh words, but still asked Lakshmana to light a fire so that she could prove her chastity.

Lakshmana lit the fire. Sita walked into the fire and said, 'I have been pure of thoughts and had not encroached upon the Lord's territory by the thought of any other man. O Lord, I have been pure but still my husband doubts me. If I, by any means—mansa, vacha and karmana (thought, speech or action)—have ever been unfaithful to my Lord, o Fire God, you can punish me but if not, you shall protect me!'

Saying so, Sita walked into the fire. The Gods from heaven said, 'Sita is serene and pure.' They pleaded Rama to take Sita out of the fire and accept her.

Confronted by Sita's chastity and purity the fire cooled down. Agnidev, the Lord of Fire, pulled her out of the flames and said to Rama, 'Sita is pure. Ravana had abducted her in the jungle because she was alone and helpless. In the Ashok Vatika, too, she was alive only by chanting your name and in the hope that you would definitely save her. Accept her, in all purity and respect. I order you not to offend her anymore or say any harsh words.' Agnidev placed Sita's hand in Rama's.

People began to celebrate Rama's victory. Lord Shiva told him, 'You have killed Ravana and this is the most auspicious thing you have done. Please proceed to Ayodhya and meet Bharata and Kaushalya. You should now take over the reins of Ayodhya in your hands.' Then, Rama told Lord Indra, 'Restore all the monkeys and bears that have been maimed or killed in this battle.'

Lord Indra rained down elixir on the monkeys and bears and they came back to life in their original form.

Rama got Mandodari married to Vibhishana, paving a prosperous life for Vibhishana's rule over Lanka and for Mandodari, who would not have to lead the life of a widow. Though Tara and Mandodari married twice in their lives, they have been given significant places as 'Sati' in Hindu mythology.

Finally, Rama chalked out his plan to reach Ayodhya. He insisted that he had to reach Ayodhya at the earliest. Vibhishana said, 'Lord, what is the hurry? Please take a bath, loosen your matted hair, rest a while, and then proceed.'

But Rama said, 'I am not feeling very good and would like to proceed to Ayodhya immediately. Bharata also must be anxious. Fourteen years are about to elapse.'

Vibhishana said, 'Do not worry! Kuber's Pushpak Viman, which Ravana had won from Kuber, is still here. It will take you to Ayodhya in a day, but I would like you to rest here for a few days.'

However, Rama insisted that he should go back. He said, 'I want to meet Bharata at the earliest. He had come to Chitrakoot to take me back, but I had disappointed him. I also wish to see my mothers at the earliest.'

Vibhishana gave in to Rama's insistence and said, 'As you wish, Lord Rama! All arrangements will be made as you desire'.

He called for the Pushpak Viman and, on Rama's instructions, offered gifts to the monkeys and bears present there and bid them farewell. Rama then asked Sugriva, Vibhishana, Jamvant, Hanuman, Angad to accompany him back to Ayodhya. All of them boarded the Puspak Viman for their journey home.

As the Pushpak Viman flew across Lanka, Rama pointed out various important locations to Sita, including the place where Ravana was cremated.

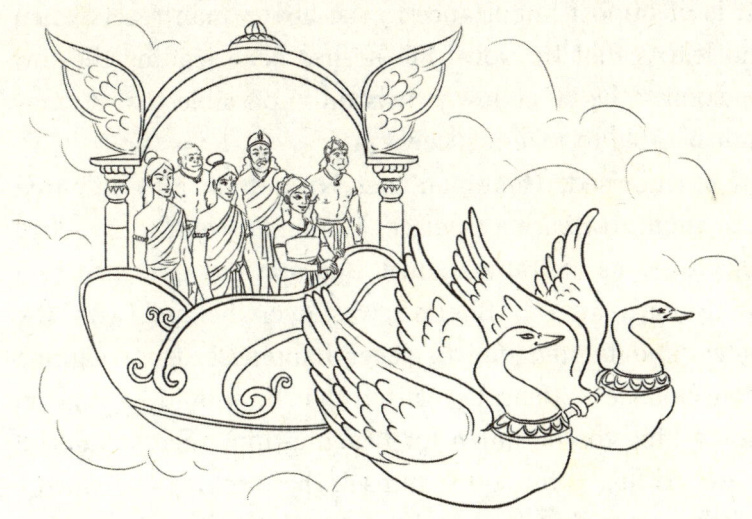

Sita said that she wished to take Tara also to Ayodhya. Rama agreed. They stopped over for a while in Kishkindha to take Tara with them. On approaching River Saryu, Rama intimated Sita, 'We have reached the banks of River Saryu. Our father's kingdom, Ayodhya, can also be seen from here. We have come back to this place after fourteen long years.' They all bowed and offered salutations to Ayodhya.

On the fifth day of the lunar cycle and at the end of fourteen years, they all reached the hermitage of Sage Bharadwaj. Bowing down to the sage, they asked about the well beings of their people and of Bharata. Rama then asked Hanuman, 'Go meet Nishadaraja and enquire about his wellbeing. Then ask him the route to Ayodhya. Go to Ayodhya and meet Bharata, but in disguise. See how he behaves and inform him that I shall be returning soon with my friends. Pay attention to his body language and expressions, when you tell him this. See how he reacts.

It is of utmost importance to see how a man reacts when he learns that the royal life he has been leading till now is soon to be taken away. It is quite possible that he may not be able to take it nicely.'

As advised, Hanuman met Nishadraja and enquired the route to Bharata's palace. Hanuman went to Ayodhya disguised as a Brahmin, met Bharata and informed him of Rama's arrival. Bharata was overwhelmed with the news and fainted due to sheer happiness. On regaining consciousness, Bharata realised that he should have given something to Hanuman for bringing him such wonderful news, although he said to himself that nothing was worthy of the news that he had brought. Even then, he offered Hanuman cows and a few women as wives. Hanuman politely refused and went back to Rama.

Bharata went and gave the good news to the queens. Hearing about Rama's arrival, all the three mothers happily gathered at Nandigram to meet and greet Rama, Lakshmana and Sita. On the other hand, Bharata happily set out to make preparations and arrangements for Rama's welcome. He went to welcome Rama about a mile from the borders of Ayodhya.

They waited impatiently for Rama's Pushpak Viman to land. They craned their necks up to get the first glimpse of the Viman. Soon, the Pushpak Viman appeared and landed where they all were standing. Rama pulled Bharata on to the Pushpak Viman and embraced him. Bharata bowed to Sita and embraced Lakshmana. Rama introduced everyone accompanying him to Bharata. He praised Vibhishana a lot and called him the epitome of virtues. Bharata addressed

Sugriva, as his fifth brother.

Bharata also praised Vibhishana and embraced him. All of them boarded the Pushpak Viman and landed at Nandigram. Rama thanked the Pushpak Viman and said, 'Please go back to Kuber.' The airplane flew back to Kuber. Rama met his mothers. He first went to Kaikeyi and touched her feet. After touching Sumitra's feet in the end, he walked up to Kaushalya to touch her feet. Shatrughana also reached the gathering and met everyone and so did Sita and Lakshmana.

Rama and Sita, after meeting their mothers, met Shatrughana. Then, they met Sage Vasishth. Bharata then said to Rama, 'You are the legitimate owner of the state, but I had to look after it for some time. Now as per your promise at Chitrakoot you have to take over. The state's royal treasury had grown ten-folds since then!'

Rama, Lakshmana and Bharata got their matted hair loosened and cut. The three brothers, along with Sita, got dressed up in royal clothes and ornaments.

# The Coronation of Lord Rama

Sage Vasishtha, conferred with Sumantra, Ashok, Vijay and Siddhartha—the ministers—and they together decided to coronate Rama as the King of Ayodhya. So that all the citizens could see their new king Rama, the procession navigated through the streets of Ayodhya. Bharata was the charioteer and Shatrughana held the umbrella over Rama. Lakshmana held the hand-fan for Rama and Sita's comfort.

Bharata asked Sugriva to arrange for the holy waters from the four directions. Sugriva entrusted Jamvant, Hanuman, Rishab and Gavey with this task of bringing the pristine water in gold pitchers (*kalashas*). Sages Vasishtha, Vamdev, Jaabali, Katyan, Suyagy, Gautam and Vijay applied the tilak on Rama's forehead. Rama was then adorned with the family crown of ancestors embedded with jewels and other ornaments. Shatrughana held a white umbrella over Rama. Pawan Dev gifted a pearl garland to Rama, which the newly-crowned King put around Sita's neck. Rama donated a number of cows, bulls and gold coins to the Brahmins. Rama gifted Sugriva a special necklace of gold and Angad an armlet. Vibhishana and the other monkeys were also blessed with gifts.

Sita took off Pawan Dev's pearl garland from her neck

and gifted it to Hanuman. Hanuman chewed one pearl from the garland, and after looking at it intently, threw it away. He repeated the sequence with all the other pearls in the garland. Everyone was surprised at Hanuman's behaviour. They asked Hanuman, 'What are you doing? Sita gave you this garland with so much affection and you have broken all its beads and threw them away.'

Hanuman replied that he was breaking every pearl and looking for his Lord Rama and Mother Sita inside the pearls, but couldn't find them. When someone asked why he was trying to find the Lord and Mother inside a pearl, Hanuman replied, 'If I did not find them in the pearls, they are of no use to me! My Lord and my Mother are always with me in my heart.'

With that, he ripped open his chest. Lord Rama and Mother Sita were visible inside. Hanuman said, 'This is all I want.' Rama and Sita were overwhelmed with emotions, and tears trickled down their cheeks.

Rama wanted to appoint Lakshmana as the crown prince, but Lakshmana refused. As such, Bharata was appointed the crown prince. After the rituals, Sugriva, Vibhishana and the others went back to their kingdoms. Hanuman stayed back with Lord Rama in Ayodhya.

The sages and hermits praised Rama for slaying the demons, but Sage Agastya appreciated Lakshmana in particular for slaying Meghnad. Out of curiosity, Rama asked the sage what was so special about slaying Meghnad. Sage Agastya said, 'Indrajeet was the bravest of the brave; there was no second to him. It was indeed a feat of bravery.'

The Pushpak Viman, which Rama had sent back to

Kuber, came back to Rama and conveyed that Kuber had said, 'This airplane was won by Ravana and since you have killed Ravana, it belongs to you now.'

It further said, 'Kuber was very pleased with what you have done. He has instructed me to be in your service.'

Rama agreed and said, 'Now you may stay in the sky, and I request you come to me whenever you are required.'

Lord Rama reigned for many long years, and also expanded his kingdom's boundaries. About his ruling period, Goswami Tulsidas has said:

*Daihik daivik bhautik tapa*
*Rama rajya nahi kahuhi vyapa*

(Rama's reign, it was believed that no one died of unnatural causes, physical or mental pain or natural calamities.)

# Sita's Exile

Rama continued to rule Ayodhya. He also went on a pilgrimage. The entire state was very happy and satisfied under his rule. Rama used to meet his informants every night to learn about issues under his rule. The chief informant was Bhadra. One night, when all the informants lined up to give their inputs, one of them remained quiet. When asked about his report, he said that he saw a washer man beating up his wife because she stayed away from her house the entire night.

The washerman had rebuked his wife and said, 'Where are you coming back from at this odd hour? Now, neither shall I let you in, nor accept you as my wife. I cannot follow Rama's footsteps, who accepted his wife Sita even after she had stayed away from him with another man for such a long time. Get out of the house.' Rama was shocked and did not return to his quarters that night. He pondered over the issue and decided that he should ask Sita to leave.

The next morning, he called his brothers and asked them to take Sita into the woods and leave her there. Bharat strongly opposed the proposal. He said that this was not an appropriate step. Then, Rama asked Lakshmana. Lakshmana, who until now had never opposed any instructions given by Rama, also refused to obey him. He said, 'Brother, I have never spoken on this matter till now, but now I shall not keep quiet. We all knew that Mother Sita was chaste. Despite that, you forced her to undergo trial by fire to prove her chastity, and you accepted her only after she passed the test. Then why this punishment now? She is also an expectant mother. Just because you heard a washer man saying something, you have decided to abandon your wife? You have made up your mind without listening to what she has to say.'

Rama said to Lakshmana, 'I do not want to listen to your argument. Either you take Sita to the forest and leave her there, or I shall end my life. Tell her that since she wanted to meet the saints, I have asked you to take her along. Then, without telling her anything, just leave her there and come back home.'

A helpless Lakshmana took Sita on a chariot along with some food, clothes and ornaments. When he reached the middle of the jungle, Lakshmana asked Sita to get down from the chariot.

Sita was surprised and she asked him, 'It is very scary out here, and I do not even know the way around! Why do you want me to get down here?' Lakshmana replied, 'Sage Valmiki's ashram is nearby. Please go there. Do not ask me anything more, I cannot tell you.'

Sita was so overcome with grief that she fainted. Lakshmana did not know what to do next. He never wanted to leave Sita behind in such a state. Just then, he heard an Akashvani (announcement from the skies): 'Lakshmana! Do not worry. You can leave Sita and go back home. She will be safe here; nothing will happen to her.' Thus, Lakshmana returned to Ayodhya.

When Sita regained consciousness, neither Lakshmana nor the chariot was anywhere to be seen. She was all alone in the forest. Her mind was flooded with emotions. She was angry and sad. She did not know what to do next. After some time, Sita tried to compose herself.

Sage Valmiki was passing by and on seeing Sita, all alone in the middle of the forest, asked her, 'Who are you?'

Sita recognized the sage and introduced herself as Janaka's daughter and Rama's wife. She told him the whole story. She said, 'I don't know why I have been abandoned by my husband. My brother-in-law has left me here without stating a reason.'

Sage Valmiki was moved. He said that Janaka is an old friend of his, and that makes her his daughter. He took her to his ashram and assured her that she shall soon be with Rama once again. Sita started living in the ashram and came to be known as Vandevi to the people.

On his way back, Lakshmana was feeling very sad, and he engaged Sumantra in conversation. He told him that he felt sad for his brother, who had been separated from his wife once again. Sumantra assuaged his feelings and said that he need not be sad, as it was destined. Even King Dasharatha was aware that circumstances would bring matters to such a juncture. Durvasa had predicted this and apprised Dasharatha of this calamity. Sumantra also was present there. This was due to the curse of Sage Bhrigu.

Sumantra further told Lakshmana that he had been sworn to secrecy about this matter, especially to the four brothers. Seeing Lakshmana's condition, Sumantra could no longer hold back the secret. However, he advised Lakshmana not to disclose it to the other brothers. They returned to Ayodhya.

After sending Sita away, Rama became very sad. He had to sacrifice his wife to keep up his ideals and the ethics of Raj Dharma (the ideals of a king). Lakshmana tried to appease him. He said, 'the truth is that whatever one accumulates gets destroyed eventually. Therefore, we should not be too attached to our women, wealth, sons or friends, because losing them would cause grief.' He told Rama to have control over his emotions.

Lakshmana went to the palace and informed the mothers about the happenings. On hearing the news, they were grief-stricken. Unable to bear the news, they died of sorrow. Rama performed their last rites.

Sita led the life of a sage at the ashram. She helped other families with their daily chores. She soon gave birth to twin boys. Sage Valmiki went to the hut where she was resting. He was mesmerized by the glowing aura of the two babies, and named them Kush and Luv.

The boys acquired their training from Valmiki. They studied and gained knowledge of the scriptures and the Vedas in the ashram itself. Valmiki taught them the art of war and the use of weapons, as well as ethics, traditions and fine arts. They were both expert archers. Having been brought up in the pure and pristine surrounding of the hermitage, they were blessed with traditional and virtuous characteristics. Valmiki scripted the story of Rama and Sita as a poetry book. Luv and Kush roamed about in the neighbouring villages and narrated this poetic story of Rama and Sita.

# The Ashwamedh Yagn

Once, Rama went to Sage Vasistha and expressed his desire to perform the Ashwamedh Yagn. Vasistha advised Bharat to make preparations for the yagn. Vibhishan, Sugriv and the others were also invited.

For the Ashwamedh Yagn, a horse was decorated in the finest livery and the empire's flag was affixed on the horse's saddle. Then, it was left to wander and the king's army followed it through whichever path it took. Whichever kingdom the horse traversed without any opposition, was assumed to have accepted the suzerainty of the empire. If the horse's path was obstructed by any king, it was an indication of war to ensue, to decide the more powerful of the two kings. After the horse had traversed the entire area without any opposition, the performing king was declared a 'Chakravarti King' (the subjugator of all). To commemorate the victory, a yagn was performed, in which the horse was given away as sacrifice.

This way, without much bloodshed, the expansion of the kingdom was accomplished. Only those who opposed were challenged to a battle.

Apart from the kings, saints and sages were also invited for the yagn. Sage Pulatsya attended the yagn along with rishi Parashar, Bhrigu, Angeera, Narad, Vyas, Agastaye and Dewal.

A messenger went to Mithila to invite King Janaka. Janaka was very pleased to see the messenger from Ayodhya and he informed his priest, Satanand, of the yagn. Satananda advised Janaka to proceed to Ayodhya. After reaching Ayodhya, Janaka was put up on the banks of the river Saryu and Bharat was entrusted with the task of making his stay comfortable in Ayodhya.

Vasistha said to Rama: 'Lord, no yagn, puja (veneration) or charitable donations are considered complete in the absence of the wife. The wife sits on the right side of the husband during such activities and plays her part. We would now need Janaki.'

Rama said: 'Lord, you are aware of everything. Now, you may do as you think is appropriate.' The sages and gurus of Ayodhya and Mithila, along with Narada, conferred amongst themselves and decided that they should place a golden idol of Sita next to Rama for the ceremony. So an idol was made and dressed in the finest clothes and ornaments. They all gathered at the site where the yagn was to be performed. The sacrificial horse for the yagn was decorated and brought to the site. 60,000 soldiers accompanied the snow white horse with black ears. It was worshiped and a note was tied to the horse.

The note read: 'A warrior from Kaushalpur (Ayodhya) is out to crush any opposition. His bravery and valour is feared, even by Lord Indra. Those who dare capture the horse shall face the consequences.'

Before the horse could be sent off, some sages came along with Sage Bhrigu and narrated the atrocities perpetrated by Lavnasur, a demon. Rama instructed Lakshmana to first go and kill Lavnasur. Shatrughana intervened and requested Rama to give him the opportunity to kill it. Rama agreed. He gave Shatrughana an arrow and said, 'Take my name and shoot this arrow. You shall have victory over all.'

Rama had gathered information about Lavnasur from Vibhishan, who told Rama, 'Kumbhsani, my cousin, is married to Madhu, the demon. Lavnasur is their son. He has pleased Lord Shiva with his penance and Lord Shiva has gifted him a Trident. As long as he has the Trident in his hand, it would be impossible to defeat him. His strength and invincibility are in that Trident. He thinks of himself as invincible and bothers everybody.'

By offering Shatrughana his powers, Rama elevated Shatrughana to a new level. Accompanied by his two sons, Subahu and Yupketu, Shatrughana left for the battle. Some texts also refer to Yupketu as Shatrughati. Lavnasur was also accompanied by his two sons, Matang and Ketu. The armies clashed with all ferocity. Subahu defeated Matang and Yupketu chopped off Ketu's arms and rendered him helpless, grovelling on the ground.

Lavnasur created an illusionary army of Gods and confused Shatrughan's army. Shatrughan destroyed this illusion with the help of Rama's arrow. Subahu struck a blow with his mace and Lavnasur fell, unconscious. Kaitabh, seeing Lavnasur unconscious, snatched the Trident from his hand and struck Yupketu, rendering him unconscious. Seeing this, Subahu shot a volley of arrows at Kaitabh, who got perturbed. Subahu helped Yupketu regain consciousness. Kaitabh then asked his brother, Jaamyak, to help, but even he was defeated. Seeing the valour of Shatrughan's sons, Jaamyak praised them and appreciated their fighting skills. Lavnasur again stepped into the battlefield, but was killed by Shatrughan. After the battle was won, Shatrughan established two beautiful cities at the site, Mathura—which he gifted to Subahu—and Vidit or Vidhisha in the west, which was gifted to Yupketu.

The yagn horse and the accompanying army now proceeded towards the south and reached Sage Valmiki's hermitage. Luv and Kush were playing there. Seeing the horse, they went near it. They read the note and tied the horse to a tree. A thousand soldiers came to that place and asked them to release the horse and go home. The twins replied, 'If you are a Kshatriya, do not beg, fight.' The soldiers tried to reason with the twins and said, 'You are young boys and do not understand the consequences of holding this horse. Do not argue and return the horse to us.'

The twins once again said, 'Have we not told you not to beg? You are a Kshatriya and are responsible for the safety of the horse. Do not beg—fight us and take it back.' Unable to take any further insults, the soldiers attacked the boys but were soon defeated. Shatrughan also reached the spot and he asked the boys to hand over the horse.

The boys asked Shatrughan, 'Who are you and where are you from? What is the meaning of the note on the horse?' Shatrughan then jokingly threatened them and said that they should now get ready with their weapons. Luv and Kush took it in their warrior spirit and said to each other, 'Now the King is trying to scare us. Has he ever heard of a lion being shooed away by the sound of claps?'

They destroyed Shatrughan's chariot and killed his charioteer and the horses. They also wounded Shatrughan. Some soldiers rushed to Rama and narrated the whole tale. Rama sent reinforcements under Lakshmana's command. Reaching the site, Lakshmana proclaimed that his family (Surya Vansh) has been the protector of the Gods and the Brahmins. He also warned the insolent boys that their words and actions were provoking anger; it would be in their favour to get out of his sight. Kush taunted Lakshmana and said, 'See your brother's state and decide. It would be in *your* favour to return home!'

Lakshmana said, 'Call your helpers' and he drew a sharp arrow. The earth shook and even 'Sheshnaag', on whose hood the earth is balanced, trembled in fear.

Arrows rained from both the sides. Luv struck a blow to Lakshmana and Lakshmana fired an arrow, meditating on the name of Rama. Luv was struck by the arrow and fell unconscious. Luv woke up and re-joined the attack. The boys cut down Lakshmana's arrows—the arrows that even Meghnad could not counter or defend himself from.

Then, Luv drew the arrow that Sage Valmiki had given to him, sanctified with mantras. This was an arrow that never missed its target. The arrow struck Lakshmana's heart and he fell unconscious. The soldiers rushed to Ayodhya and once again narrated the happenings to Rama. Bharat said that they were being punished by Lord Brahma for abandoning Sita.

Rama derided Bharat and said that if he was scared of fighting, he (Bharat) might as well take care of the yagn here and Rama would go and end the battle. Bharat was embarrassed and humiliated but said nothing. Rama instructed him to take Angad, Hanuman, Jamvant and Sugriv along and finish the job. Bharat followed Rama's instructions and reached the site. He said to Vibhishan, 'Go with Sugriv, Hanuman and Angad.' Vibhishan did as he was told. Seeing Angad, Kush said, 'Everyone is aware of your strength. You first got your father killed, then kept your mother at another man's house, and today you dare to come here?'

Angad became furious and rushed with a huge rock towards Kush. Kush destroyed the rock with his arrow. He then shot five arrows at Angad and the others. Then, Hanuman, Jamvant and Sugriv rushed to attack with boulders and rocks, but the twins reduced these weapons to rubble. All the monkeys were subjugated. Bharat shot an arrow at Luv. He was struck in the heart and he fell down, unconscious. Kush retaliated with a volley of 100 arrows at Bharat. Bharat was struck and lost consciousness. Kush helped Luv regain consciousness and hugged him. Four messengers, who were watching the on-going battle from a distance, went back to Rama and informed him of what had happened. Rama left the yagn midway, gathered his army and marched to the battle site.

Rama, on seeing the beautiful hermit boys, signalled them to come closer. He said, 'Tell me the name of your father and mother. Who are you and where are you from? You have won a great battle.'

The twins retorted, 'Pick up your arms and fight.' Rama said, 'Without knowing your name and your place of origin, I shall not fight you.'

Luv and Kush then introduced themselves, saying 'Our mother's name is Sita and she is the daughter of King Janaka. Sage Valmiki has brought us up and our names are Luv and Kush. We do not know our father's name or his clan.'

Rama was glad that he had not hurt them and had instead coerced them into introducing themselves. He thought to himself that it would not be appropriate to fight them. Rama then told the boys that his warriors would challenge them, but he would not fight them. Rama asked Nal, Neel, Angad, Sugriv and the other mighty apes to take up the challenge. Meanwhile, Luv stepped forward and derided Vibhishana, 'Fool, you deserted your brother and joined the enemy's camp. You married your brother's wife, the woman whom you would have called 'mother' so many times. Are these your virtues and beliefs? You should be ashamed of yourself.' Vibhishan was humiliated and angry. He rushed towards Luv with his mace to attack him. Luv shot an arrow and broke his mace into pieces. Vibhishana then threw his spear at Luv. The brothers not only destroyed the spear but also everything else that came their way. Luv shot Sugriva in the heart, and he was flung seven leagues away. Kush slammed Jamvant into the ground and tied him up. They then tied up Hanuman and kept him near the horse. Kush asked Luv to wait for him near the horse and went to meet Rama, who was sound asleep in his chariot. Kush did not wake him up, nor thought it proper to strike him. So he just returned and let him sleep.

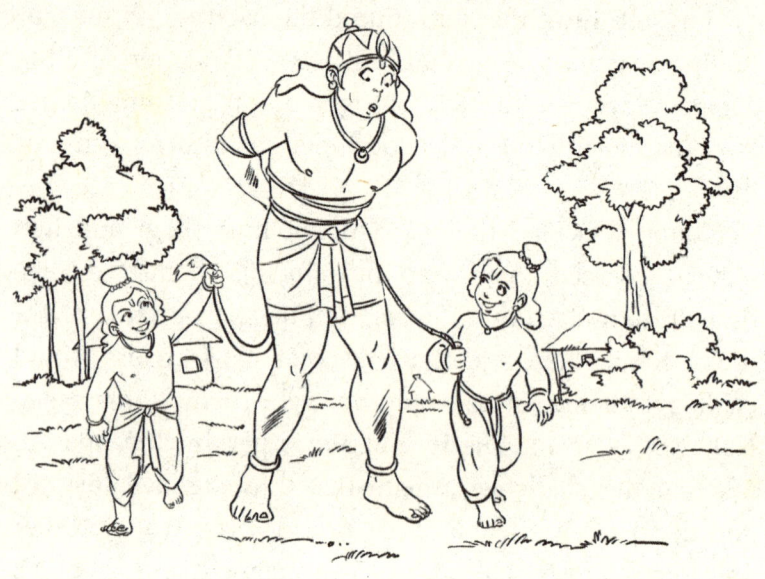

The brothers gathered all the weapons, clothes and ornaments worn by the soldiers and went back to their ashram with Hanuman and Jamvanta. They lay their spoils in front of their mother and bowed down to her. Kush said to his mother, 'See, what a beautiful horse we have brought and also a monkey and a bear. I shall play with them.' She was mesmerized at the sight of the horse and did not hear what Kush was saying. She saw the standard of Ayodhya flying on the horse. On the flag of Ayodhya, there was the image of a Kovidar tree with bright stems. She then noticed Hanuman and Jamvanta tied up. Valmiki rushed to find out what was happening. Sita then pleaded with Hanuman and Jamvanta to pardon her children and untied them. Hanuman touched Sita's feet and sought her blessings. Tears rolled down his cheeks as he called out to Sita. Whether these tears were of happiness or of regret, is not known.

Sita then introduced Hanuman to Luv and Kush and said, 'He is an ardent devotee of your father. He has been very helpful to your father in very many difficult situations. He is like your elder brother. Bow down to him and take his blessings.' Luv and Kush did as they were told. Hanuman hugged them tightly, pulling them close to his heart. She then admonished Luv and Kush and said that what they had done today was the most disgraceful thing to do. They had defeated Rama, Lakshmana, Bharata and Shatrughana in battle and had rendered them soulless. Lord Brahma had widowed her. She would now become a Sati.

Valmiki assuaged Sita's fear and they all went to the site of the battle. Valmiki was very happy with the feat of the boys and the skill with which they defeated the army. Valmiki bowed down to Lord Rama and introduced the boys as his sons. Rama hugged them and Valmiki narrated the whole story. Bharat, Lakshmana and Shatrughana also regained consciousness and seeing Sita, bowed down and touched her feet. She then introduced the twins to them and the uncles blessed and embraced their nephews. Rama was once again overcome with emotions and hugged his sons tightly. Luv and Kush touched his feet.

Rama had seen many unfavourable situations and conditions in his life, and he had faced them valiantly and had come out victorious. He made every effort to taste victory, and was successful. Taking the right decision at the right time made him a successful strategist. He displayed good diplomacy by taking the relatives of his enemies under his wings to buttress his efforts and endeavours. To win over Sugriv, he killed Bali and to defeat Ravana, he won over Vibhishan. But now, an act that had contradicted his ideals led to his humiliation and defeat by his own sons. These are the finer points of this episode in the Ramayana.

After everyone met Luv and Kush, Rama stepped towards Sita and said, 'Come Sita, let us go home.' But Sita stopped him midway and said, 'Stop there, do not try to come any closer. You sent me to the forest just on the hearsay of a washerman. Your duties and responsibility as a king were more important than my affection and feelings for you. You disowned me. So what made you change your mind now? Let me stay where I am!'

Rama said, 'No, I know that I have caused a lot of pain to you. Please forget everything and let us go home.' But Sita refused. She said, 'I do not want anyone to blame you for not upholding your principles in future. This will make you weak and your decision will be driven by emotions. Now, if you force me to go with you, I shall ask Mother Earth to take me, and I shall sleep there forever.'

Rama then begged Sita, and pleaded, 'No, my dear Sita, please do not utter such harsh words. Your place is next to me on the throne.' Sita refused, saying, 'You had once abandoned me. Then, on what grounds are you taking me back now? How can you say for sure if you were right then or are right now? If you were right then, they how will you explain to your subjects why you are taking me back to the palace in the first place? I do not want you to be embarrassed, since you would fail to justify your actions.

You are challenging your own actions. Our sons have to bear the fruits of our separation and the consequences of your folly. Now, I wish that Mother Earth would open up and take me in so that I may sleep in her lap forever.'

Sita stood with folded hands and prayed to Mother Earth, 'If I have been true and only seen my Lord in thoughts, words, deeds and actions (Mansa, Vacha and Karmana) and if I have never ever thought of any other man in his place—if I have been always with him in good and bad times—o Mother Earth, please open up and take me.'

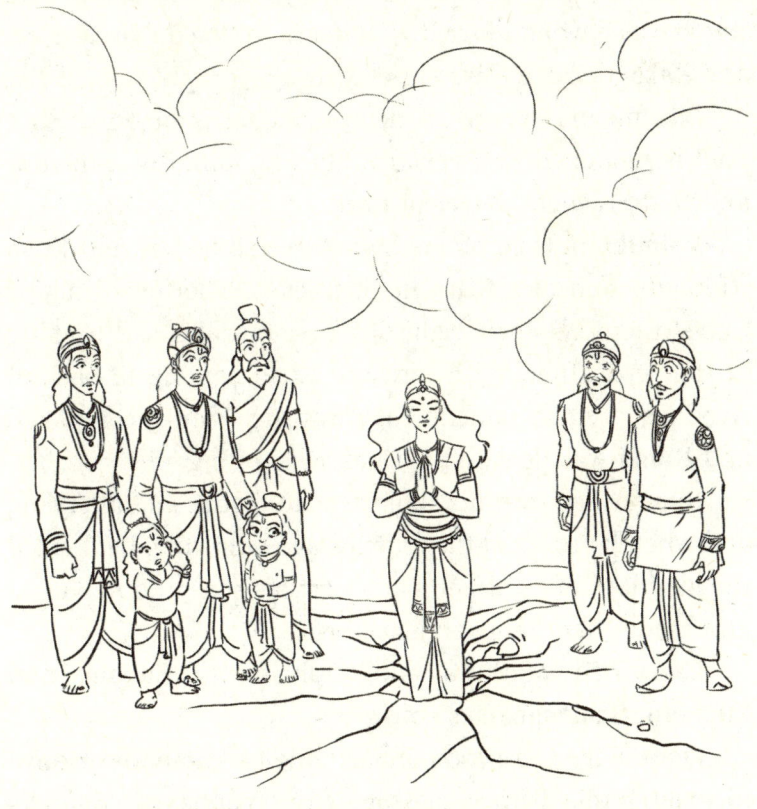

The earth started to tremble. Lakshmana, who had been a part of the entire, sad incident, could not take it anymore. Ever since he had left Sita back in the jungle, he had been unable to forgive himself. He wanted to end his life, but had stopped himself from doing so. Now, once again, he was overwhelmed with emotions and could no longer hold back his feelings. He rose from the earth in his true form, as Sheshnaag, and carried a golden throne with him. He asked Sita to sit on the throne and slithered into the netherworld. The earth smoothened and everyone was stunned and mesmerized at what had just happened. Rama was beyond himself, with tears rolling down his face, and Lakshmana too was grief stricken.

Sita means 'furrow', a deep line that is made when a field is ploughed (*hal rekha*). Sita was found in a furrow, and that is where she went back.

Valmiki and the others bade farewell to Luv and Kush with affection and tears in their eyes. They were happy to see them get their rightful place, but also sad because of the separation. With Luv and Kush coming to back to Ayodhya, the Ashwamedh Yagn was successfully completed and Rama was declared a 'Chakravarti king'.

Rama ruled over his subjects with justice and affection, and when he reached the fourth stage of his life, he divided the kingdom in eight parts amongst his sons and nephews, and made them independent kings.

He gifted Mathura and Vidhisha to Subahu and Yupketu, Shatrughana's sons.

Once, Sage Gargi, son of Sage Angira, came to Ayodhya to meet Rama with a message from Yudhajeet, Bharat's maternal uncle. The message said, 'On the banks of the river Sindhu lies the land ruled by the Gandharva King Sailush and his 30 million sons. Send an army and conquer this land and establish a new empire. Taksh and Pushkal, Bharat's sons, may be seated on the throne, and they shall rule under my patronage.'

Bharat set out with an army from Ayodhya. He was joined by Yudhajeet on the way and together, they attacked the kingdom of the Gandharvas. After a fierce battle, Bharat shot the Sarvat, and all the Gandharvas were killed. He then carved out two kingdoms from the land—Takshila, under Taksh or Sutaksh's rule, and Pushkalavat, under Pushkal. Bharat stayed with them for a few days, to guide and organize their rule, and then returned to Ayodhya.

After Bharat's and Shatrughan's sons were crowned, Rama told Lakshmana that now it was time for his sons to settle down. He should look for a beautiful empire, bereft of any hurdles or obstacles, which could be handed over to his sons. Bharat suggested that Kaarupath was indeed a beautiful place and Mahatma Angad (Lakshmana's son, not to be confused with Vali's son) should be made the king of the scenic kingdom. He also suggested creating Chandrakanta, a kingdom for Chandrakant or Chandraketu, the second son of Lakshmana. This was another beautiful place with a scenic and a healthy ambiance.

Accepting Bharat's suggestion, Rama subjugated Kaarupath and named its capital Angdiya. Angad was crowned as the king of this state. Chandraketu had a muscular and bulky body like the *mallah*s, or boatmen, and so his kingdom was created out of the boatmen's territory and named Chandrakanta. Lakshmana accompanied Angad to his kingdom while Bharat accompanied Chandrakant to his. They helped the young kings settle down and learn the art of ruling and presiding over their subjects. They stayed with them for a year and returned to Ayodhya. The Northern territory of Kaushal was placed under Luv's rule, whereas the southern territory was given to Kush. Carved out of the Vindhyachals, Kushavati was created for Kush and Shravasti was created for Luv.

After dividing the kingdom amongst the eight sons of the family, Rama, Lakshmana, Bharat and Shatrughan lived together in the palace, leading a simple, ascetic life.

# The Journey to the Heavens

The four brothers spent a long life in this world, until Yamraj thought that any further delay would spoil the equation of life and death. He thought of sharing his thoughts with Lord Rama. He disguised himself as a sage and came to Ayodhya. He met Rama and said that he wished to discuss the cycle of life and death with him.

Rama said to Lakshmana, 'I have a very important issue to discuss with Yamraj and do not wish to be disturbed. I would also like that no one overhears our conversation.'

When this conversation was taking place, Hanuman was not around. He had gone to the netherworld to look for Rama's ring. So Rama asked Lakshmana to stand guard with strict instructions that no one should be allowed to enter the chamber. If someone did, Rama would punish the intruder with death.

Lakshmana stood guard as Rama and Yamraj continued with their talks. Rama asked Yamraj what he wished to discuss. He was eager to hear him out.

Yamraj said that he had come with a message from Lord Brahma. Yamraj said, 'You are an ideal man, Lord Vishnu, the protector of all. You had been incarnated in this human form to kill Ravana. The task for which you had been incarnated has come to an end, and so your time is over.'

Rama said to Yamraj, 'I am ready to leave this world.'

When this conversation between Lord Rama and Yamraj was going on, Sage Durvasa arrived at the palace and demanded to meet Rama. The guards took him to Lakshmana, who requested the sage to rest and wait for the Lord, as Rama was busy. He could meet him as soon as he was free.

Durvasa was infamous for his fiery temper. Even the slightest reason could send him into a fit of rage. He chided Lakshmana, 'You are asking me to wait. This is impossible. Either you go inside and tell Rama that I have come to meet him, or let me go inside immediately. Otherwise, I shall burn this universe.'

Lakshmana was in a dilemma! If he went inside, Lord Rama would execute him, and if he did not, Durvasa would burn the universe down. In either scenario, his end was certain. So he decided to step into Rama's chamber and accept death at his hands.

He said to Durvasa, 'Please wait. I shall inform Lord Rama of your arrival.' Duravasa agreed and Lakshmana went inside. Seeing Lakshmana, Rama was perturbed. He said, 'What have you done, Lakshmana! Now I will have to...'

Lakshmana said, 'Lord, if I had not come inside, Durvasa would have burnt the universe down. So, I thought I might as well come in. At least, the universe would be saved and only I would have to die.' Rama accepted Lakshmana's justification and said that he would now meet Durvasa, as he was finished with Yamraj. Yamraj also took his leave, saying that his errand was over and he would now return to his abode.

Rama met Durvasa and asked him his reason for the visit. Sage Durvasa said, 'I have completed a thousand years of penance and have come straight to you. I am hungry; serve me food—whatever is ready and available.' Rama arranged for a sumptuous meal for the sage.

After having his meal, Durvasa went back to his hermitage. Now Rama was left wondering—how could he kill his own brother, Lakshmana! He said that as he had already had a word with Yamraj, the question of punishment did not hold.

Lakshmana said, 'Brother, to uphold virtues, you banished Sita. Then why are you not willing to show the same fortitude and idealistic approach for me? Please do not go back on your words and disgrace the family.'

Rama called a priest for his advice and narrated the whole incident. The priest advised Rama to disown Lakshmana. Doing so would be equivalent to death for Lakshmana. He should not break his vow and disgrace the family traditions. Rama agreed and did as was told.

After hearing this, Lakshmana did not say a word to anyone. He quietly went out of the palace and reached the banks of the river Saryu. He bowed to the river with folded hands and walked to the middle of the river. He immersed himself completely in the water, and when he reappeared on the surface, it was in the form of Sheshnaag (his original self). He dived into the water again and never came back up.

Rama was heart-broken when he saw Lakshmana immersing himself in the water of Saryu, never to rise again. Lakshmana had been with him through thick and thin—from protecting Vishwamitra's yagn from the demons to the battle with Ravana.

Sita's parting words were still ringing in his ears. Yamraj's words about his purpose were also provoking Rama to take the final step. Ultimately, he decided to take leave of this world. Accompanied by his brothers Bharat and Shatrughana, he arrived at the banks of the river Saryu to immerse himself in the water and accept eternal sleep.

When Rama, along with his brothers, went to the river, Hanuman, Sugriva, Vibhishana and others also accompanied them. They all wanted to go along with him on the final journey. Rama took Bharata, Shatrughana, and Sugriv and the other monkeys with him, but he left behind Vibhishana, Jamvanta, Hanuman, Maind and Dwividh. He told Vibhishana, 'You shall stay on earth as long as humanity exists.' He said to Hanuman, 'You have vowed to stay till eternity. Do not break the vow. As long as there are people to listen to my story, you shall stay here by my order and propagate the same.' Hanuman assured him and said that he would stay as long as the Rama Katha is narrated and heard.

Rama told the others to inhabit earth until the universe itself ends due to a calamity after Kal Yug. Out of the five, Jamvant, Maind and Dwividh would either die or be killed between the Dwapar and Kal Yugs.

The other monkeys left with Rama for his heavenly abode. When Rama immersed himself in the water of the Saryu, he recited the Vedas, and through his divine powers, assimilated Bharat unto him. Shatrughana also merged with him in the form of a lotus.

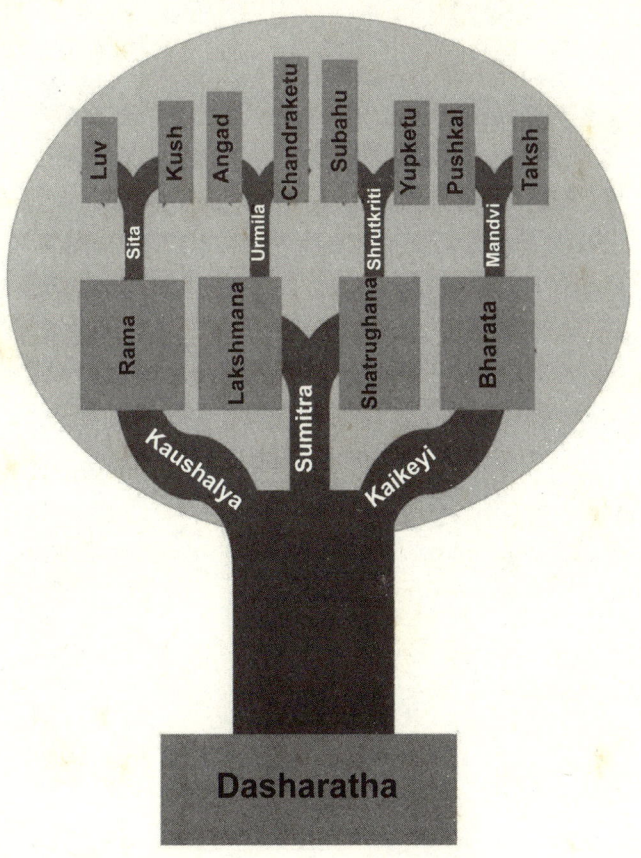

The Journey to the Heavens